Food, Africa, and the Pursuit of Contentedness

Mark Schultz

Printed in the United States of America

Published by Backwood Basics Press

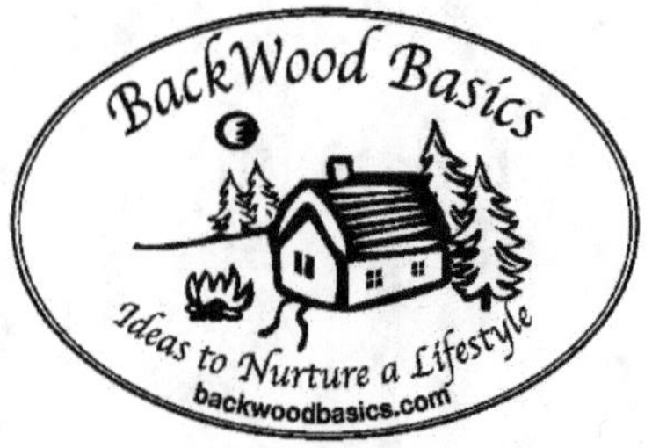

backwoodbasics.com

ISBN: 9798596812039

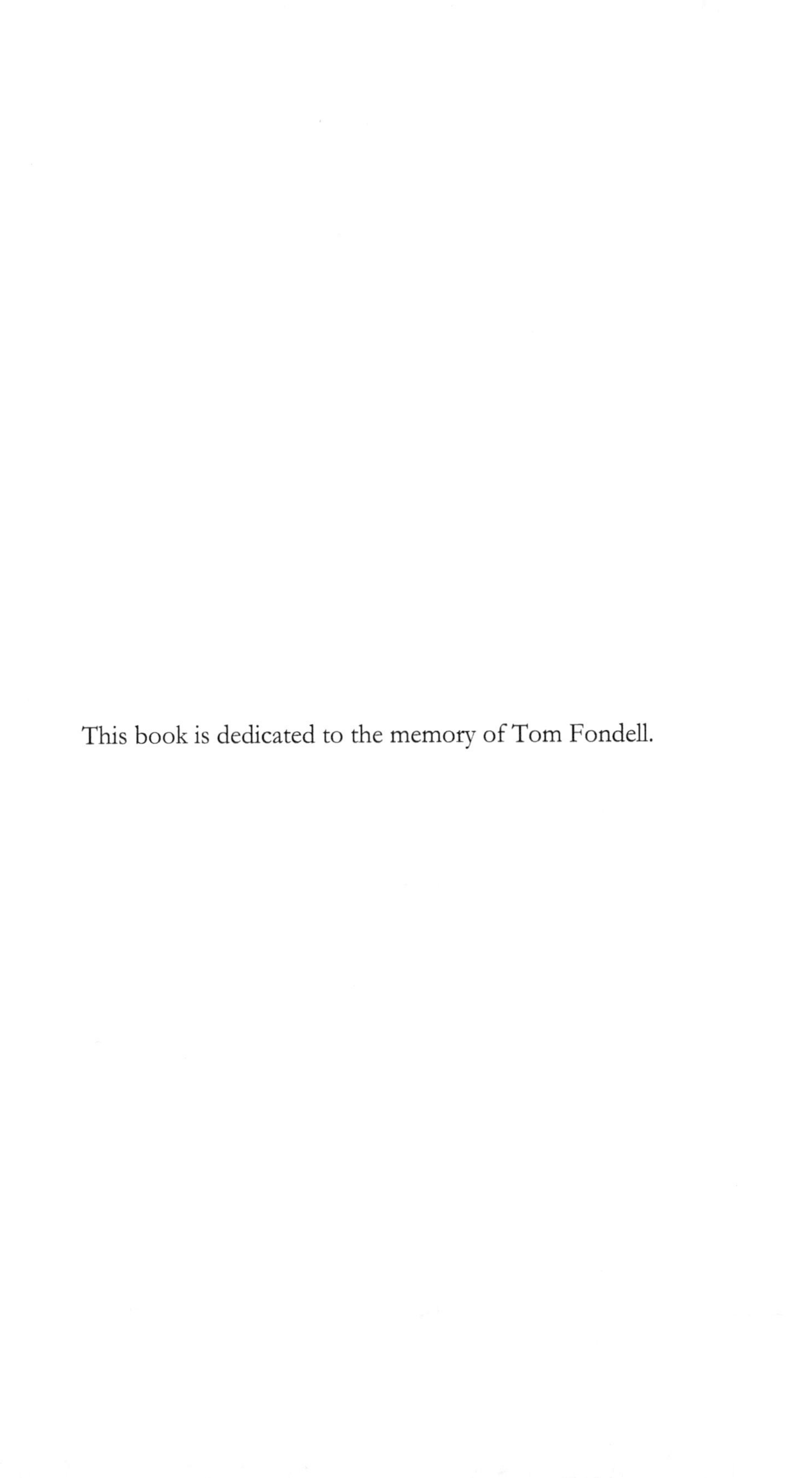

This book is dedicated to the memory of Tom Fondell.

INTRODUCTION

I had an introduction all written for this book; or at least I thought I had. That was before my daughter, Sarah, and I flew down to SW Florida to retrieve my almost 90-year-old mother, and bring her back to Bemidji, Minnesota, where we live. Sarah works at an Assisted Living facility, where my mother was to reside, so she could then come out to our place for regular visits, and, as she put it "eat lots of fat". Mom loves a good, fatty beef brisket or a picnic ham, or pretty-much anything fatty that comes off the Weber or out of the smoker. This was in mid-March of 2020. We had exactly 3 days of freedom to visit before the lock-down. Besides my mother having to spend her 90th birthday by herself, much of the whole world came to a screeching halt.

Folks who know more about it than I do will be writing about this pandemic. I want to focus on how it has affected some of our attitudes toward diet, priorities, and lifestyles, which is basically what this book is about. My pre-pandemic introduction focused on industrial agricultural practices, and how they strive to subdue and conquer nature. Instead of partnering with nature to grow food in healthy, living soil, most of our food is grown in dead or dying soil, using chemicals that further degrade the soil and turn our food into nutrient-deficient, chemically-dependent, sorry stuff that is making us sick. The way I see it, we are just smart enough to get ourselves into deep trouble. Unintended consequences are around every corner. Whether it's the use of insecticides, herbicides, fungicides, genetically engineered organisms, or preservatives, they all have their own unintended consequences. None of us, not even the white lab-coated chemists who create them, know just what goes on at the cellular level, or how our cells will respond to the faulty information being fed to them by these chemicals.

On the flipside are the growing number of farmers who are now practicing Regenerative Farming. These are farmers who are partnering with nature, instead of with the chemists in white lab coats, to grow food. They are nurturing healthy soil by going no-till, planting diverse cover crops, keeping the soil covered, and incorporating livestock through mob-grazing. By nourishing the soil, they are feeding, and providing a home for, the decomposers, which then feed the plants, and sequester tons of carbon into the soil in the process. It is said that if enough farmers would practice Regenerative Farming, we could sequester enough carbon to bring CO_2 levels in the atmosphere back to pre-industrial levels. It just may be the only thing that will save us from ourselves.

Pushing the pause button had some interesting results. Garden seed supplies ran out. Potting soil, chicken feed, day old chicks, fishing tackle, bullets, and canning lids were all in short supply. State Parks had record attendances, as newbie campers took to the woods. This new-found interest in the world of self-reliance may have caused hardships for us veteran growers, but it was heartening to see, none-the-less. I understand that we are a crisis-oriented society, and that our memories are short. But some of it might stick.

As exciting as this novel interest in self-reliance was, I found the long lines of vehicles behind the drive-up windows at fast food joints disheartening. Instead of our leaders declaring industrial food as essential, why were they not advising folks to eat wholesome, clean, locally grown foods that would nourish our bodies, restore local economies, and boost our immune systems? What, besides starch, is in those fast-food French fries? Being grown in dead soil, they are likely laced with herbicides, fungicides, insecticides, and even a growth inhibitor to keep them from sprouting. Most of these chemicals are endocrine disruptors, which are chemicals that mimic, replace, or disrupt the hormones or enzymes that regulate cellular functions. How our government can allow these chemicals to be unleashed into our air, water, soil and our food is beyond me. Why in the world would we knowingly ingest chemicals that can make our microbiomes go haywire, and trick our cells into doing things they don't want to do, like growing tumors? I think Hagrid's advice to Harry, Ron, and Hermione in *Harry Potter and the Sorcerer's Stone* would also be sound advice for Big Ag and Big Food: *"You're meddling in things that ought not to be meddled in. It's dangerous!"* Well said, Hagrid.

As futile as it seems, it's still important to know that we have a vote in how our food is grown. Our Department of Agriculture (USDA) may be cozy with Big Ag; and the handful of food giants that run the show seem to have unstoppable power. But just a decade ago Regenerative Farming was not even part of the vocabulary of mainstream farming. Now, 2 Minnesota-based biggies, Cargill and General Mills, are talking about no-till farming, and reducing the use of herbicides. This is only because consumers have expressed concern about glyphosate in their breakfast cereal. Even industry giants fear the loss of market share. Shareholders don't like to see it, so voting with our dollars, by buying clean food grown in living soil, might get more attention than one would think.

A final thought on this pandemic is one that we may find unsettling. We have become so distanced from nature that we start to think that we can depend on the chemists in white lab coats to fix everything. But lurking in the backs of our minds is the unnerving thought that maybe nature is the boss after all. What if we really can't conquer and subdue nature? What if we tick nature off to the point where, like a patient parent who finally snaps, she says: *"That's enough!"* Pandemics teach us that nature is, and always will be, the boss. Some say that we are going to kill the planet with our abuses. I don't think so. I think that the planet, and the natural world, will be just fine. There just may not be any of us humans running around to know it.

On that cheerful note, I want to take you into the heart of Africa, where Peggy and I met, and where we learned so much about what is important in life, and how our experiences there have shaped our lives here. But first, I want to start at the beginning, at least at my beginning, for perspective.

THE TIME OF GREAT CHANGE

I grew up in one of those new $12,000 homes that sprouted from the potato fields fringing the northern Minneapolis city limits. In 1956, which is the year I was born, my parents moved from the farming community of Willmar, Minnesota, to what would become Brooklyn Center. My dad got a job running the bottling machine at Ewald Brothers Dairy in North Minneapolis and worked there until the dairy closed in the late 1960s.

I call this the *Time of Great Change* because I saw this as the time when meal preparation passed from Mom to food corporations. I recall the Ewald Brothers milk truck pulling into our driveway and the uniformed driver emerging with his metal basket that contained our order. During his previous visit, he'd picked up the list that Mom had left for him —along with the rinsed, empty glass bottles—in the cooler on our back steps. Since Mom was generally home, there was little fear of these dairy products being left in the box for too long. I also recall going with my parents to nearby Robbinsdale to do our shopping in our massive blue 1957 Plymouth with the big fins on the back, since our neighborhood was too new to have any nearby stores.

I could reminisce for pages about my life as a first-generation, free-range suburban kid. It truly was a magical time of perceived innocence and safety, from the Tonka truck construction projects to the best entertainment a suburban kid could hope for—the burn barrel. We were pretty much a monoculture of skinny little white-haired kids. Most of our dads were World War II veterans, and none of them ever really talked about the war. It was enough for them to know that, through their efforts and sacrifices, their kids saw their little world as one of innocence and safety. We were not without diversity, however. On our block alone, there were *two* Catholic kids.

The Time of Great Change was born when television sets started showing up in our living rooms. Saturday morning cartoons soon became mandatory viewing, and they were of excellent quality back then. Interspersed between episodes of *Looney Tunes* (they were the best), *Milton the Monster*, *George of the Jungle*, and other classics, were ads for some really cool toys and sugar-fortified cereals. I *had* to have that cereal, so I would go grocery shopping with Mom. She would drop me off in the cereal aisle, do her shopping, and pick me and my selection(s) up before heading to the checkout. As soon as we got home, I would have the entire contents of the box poured into a bowl so I could extract the toy that was inevitably at the bottom of the box.

Mom, on the other hand, would shop for hamburger on sale, and everything that would accompany the hamburger. Hamburger formed the foundation of most of our meals, generally in the form of *hotdishes* (the rest of the world outside of Minnesota calls them *casseroles*, which are the containers in which one bakes a hotdish). Like most parents in our neighborhood, mine grew up on farms and brought their farm meal traditions with them to the new suburbs. This was not to continue much longer, however.

The television/food corporation marriage was an unprecedented success. Mine became the first generation ever in the history of mankind to spend its formative years consuming a diet so high in processed foods and refined carbohydrates. A mom-made meal had, at its core, love for the family that she was feeding. Food was selected, prepared, and served with concern for the health and well-being of her family. But Mom was only human. On occasion, even she succumbed to the seductive ads for convenience foods, and would occasionally cut loose and serve us TV dinners. We could not, of course, actually watch TV while we were eating our TV dinners, like the families did on the commercials; that was far too decadent. But they were a treat nonetheless. The food in them was truly awful, but it was so much fun to bake and eat right out of a foil tray, with each entrée in its own compartment. The poor-quality, commercially prepared food was heavily dosed with salt, sugar, and fat, which made it taste darn good to us kids. Of course, if the same food had been served to us from a pot on the stove, we would have turned our noses up at it. The food industry was on to something, though. Not only could they get kids to beg for expensive, lousy food, but they could get people like my mother to buy it.

From this point on, it was off-to-the-races for the corporations. Soon, Mom had to get a job outside the home to help pay for the convenience items that the ads on television enticed us to need; and since she was working, someone else was going to have to make convenient foods for her to serve to her family. Soon, we all had new appliances and window air conditioners, and we would sit around and brag about who had the most Btus (although none of us had a clue what a Btu was). Folks flocked to the growing suburbs to get the jobs that they needed to pay for those convenience items. Soon, the remaining farmland fringing the Twin Cities was transformed into more suburbs. Roads were widened and lined with new shopping centers, car dealerships, banks, and food joints—lots of food joints.

When the corporations became big and powerful enough to do so, they convinced our government that the best way to teach kids how to appreciate processed, factory-made food was to introduce it as part of the curriculum, during the lunch hour, in our public schools. If anyone doubts that the food giants have power, remember that our lawmakers in Washington have decreed that the thin coat of tomato sauce on factory-made pizza is now considered a serving of vegetables for our children. We may think of it as just another funny story coming out of Washington but declaring pizza a vegetable has kept it on the school lunch menu.

I know it was a bit of an illusion, but the 50s seemed to me to be a time of moderation, with moderate incomes, exercise, work, leisure, and meals. Our lives seemed to be on a steady course, kind of like an airplane flying sedately at a constant altitude. Then, along came television, the power of advertising, and corporate-structured businesses convincing us that we needed more of their products and, of course, more money to pay for those products. A snowball effect was set in motion that seemed to squash everything in its path, things like family relationships, virtues, marriages, and our faith. Our nation became more greed-driven, with the corporate world growing richer and more powerful every year. Our society became less like an airplane cruising at a steady altitude and more like a rocket, climbing higher and faster while consuming tons of fuel. Our health care system now has an obesity epidemic on its hands that will almost certainly bankrupt it, and we are losing topsoil at an astonishing rate. But everything that goes up must come down. I think it is time to strap on a parachute and get off this ride. It's time to visit Africa.

INTO AFRICA

I graduated from Bemidji State University in north-central Minnesota in 1980, with a degree in environmental studies. By then I was already advancing in my career as a dock boy at an area campground. By my third season, I was pulling down a cool $100 per week, up substantially from my entry-level salary of $65 per week (which included room and board and free use of the boats). During the off-season, I supplemented my income by cutting firewood. Bemidji in the early 1980s was a place where a rural newspaper delivery position was considered a highly competitive job.

I needed a change but going back down to the now-bustling Twin Cities was not an option. Joining the Peace Corps had been lurking as a wild, exotic thought for some time. This thought had been planted by a lust to see the world, tales from adventuresome friends, and a neighbor in Bemidji who had served as a Peace Corps volunteer in Cameroon. I finally convinced myself that I was considering it for the work experience. After two years, I could come back to Bemidji and just walk right into that paperboy job.

I thought maybe I wanted to go to the South Pacific and raise milkfish. I had no clue what a milkfish was, but then, I didn't know what a tilapia was either. I could either get on the waiting list for a post in the South Pacific or take a fisheries position that was available right away in the Central African Republic. Wow. Africa. I had seen a few *Tarzan* movies, but that was it for my education

"

about Africa. It was time to visit the library to bone up on the Central African Republic.

It's strange, but I do not recall what made me finally decide to drive to the Peace Corps recruiting office in downtown Minneapolis on that winter day; I just recall that it was snowing big, soft, fluffy flakes of snow. In my experience, God does not direct our actions. First off, I believe that it is more likely angels have been delegated to watch over their assigned humans. From them, we receive gentle nudges in one direction or another—whispers, not commands. I have felt myself being nudged and have, thankfully, responded (at least some of the time). The decision to drive to the recruiting office led (eventually) to the existence of my family, the people I cannot imagine life without. Peggy, who grew up in the spectacular Hudson River Valley about thirty-five miles north of New York City, was still a year out from responding to her nudges.

I flew out of the Minneapolis airport on April 7, 1982 for Norman, Oklahoma, and ten weeks of intensive fisheries training at the University of Oklahoma. Also standing in line was my soon-to-be best buddy for the next two and a half years, Tom Fondell. It was obvious that we were both embarking on the same adventure. We were both dragging massive duffel bags, and were flanked by rather apprehensive-looking parents. Together, we were to become the legendary *Basse-Kotto Boys*. But I'm getting ahead of myself.

Tom, Pete, Mac, Rebecca, and I completed our training in Oklahoma, and arrived in Bangui, the capital of the Central African Republic (CAR), in July of 1982. The five of us had been through the type of training session that creates either inseparable bonds or insanity. Nothing would separate us—or so we thought. Tom and I were, of course, from Minnesota. Mac was from California, a place I envisioned was nothing but beaches and surfers. Pete hailed from New Jersey, a place I had no concept of (and still don't). Our group of 30 some trainees was destined for several different countries, both in Africa and in Central America.

The staff therefore tried to house us together by country, so we could begin our bonding process. The 4 of us guys were together in our own mobile home, since our lodging was in a trailer park. In Oklahoma! In the summer! I may not have been very well-traveled, but I at least knew about tornados. While the Californian and the New Jerseyite slept soundly through wild thunderstorms, Tom and I had the good sense to huddle next to the radio, as our strapped down trailer shuddered in the wildest storms I had ever witnessed. Rebecca hailed most recently from Colorado and, being female, had to be housed with other females going to other countries. But the 5 of us still roamed together as a pack when we could get away with it.

We flew from Oklahoma City to New York City, where we boarded a flight to Paris. My first time on a jetliner was going to Oklahoma, and my first-ever view of an ocean was while crossing it. Then we had a layover in Paris, of all places. Well, I wanted to see the world, and here it was. Rebecca had studied in Paris and was fluent in French, so she took her charges under her wing. She brought us to a sidewalk café where we drank beer with lemon in it, and then we went to see the Eiffel Tower, where we all promptly fell asleep on the lawn.

We boarded our flight to Bangui, which had a layover in Rome. We didn't get off the plane, but I still counted it as a trip to Rome. Somewhere over northern Africa, our DC-10 was embroiled in a fierce thunderstorm. The massive aircraft dropped like a rock several times. Food trays went flying and passengers screamed, but I was too dumb to be scared. I was so unfamiliar with flying that I assumed that this was a typical occurrence. I later learned that flying into places like Bangui can be risky because the airports are not equipped with radar (or electricity). Planes must rely on onboard radar to anticipate storms—or other aircraft. But by then it was too late to be scared.

Landing in Bangui was a bit unreal, but some of that may have been due to jet lag. Stepping off the plane, we were hit with Africa.

There was the oppressive heat and humidity, but most overwhelming was the acrid, permeating smell of wood smoke. Even in the capital, wood was the primary cooking fuel, and this was not the aromatic pine scent that I was accustomed to in Minnesota. The smell of burning tropical hardwood is strong and pungent, like burning the punks we used for lighting fireworks. But we were still all together, and we would be until we arrived at our language training facility in M'Baiki, an area of lush rainforest southwest of Bangui. Here, our fellowship was about to suffer its first disruption.

We were met by the language professor who evaluated our French proficiency levels to determine which class we would be placed in. Rebecca, as I mentioned, was fluent, so she was placed in an advanced class. When the professor spoke to me in French, I smiled and explained that I only spoke German. In fourth through sixth grade at Northport Elementary, our teachers would wheel in the big black-and-white television set every day at 2 p.m., turn on Channel 2, and we would spend a half hour chatting in German with Frau Oplicht. I even took German in seventh grade. When he then rattled off some gibberish, I shook my head, asking what language he had spoken. He said, *"German."*

It turns out Tom, Mac, and Pete were no more proficient in French (or German) than I was, so at least the four of us remained together. Each of the classes were named for a river in Africa, and it stung a bit when we were told that our class was the French word for *Nile*. We were to be the *Nils*. The CAR had one thing going for it that many other African nations did not: one unifying national language. The Sango were a fishing tribe and, historically, the primary traders of goods. Their language became the trade language and eventually the national language, unlike countries such as Zaire, which had over 200 tribal dialects. We not only had to learn French, the official language, but Sango as well. We still got to see Rebecca outside of class, but the problem was this rule called *total immersion,* which meant that we could only speak in

French or Sango. Rebecca soon tired of looking at 4 mute, blank faces, and left us Nils to fend for ourselves.

Sango was a fun language to mess around with. Its *Me-Tarzan-You-Jane* simplicity made it seem easy to learn. Many volunteers mastered it. I did not, despite hiring a student in Mobaye as a once-a-week tutor. Our struggles with the languages became a source of entertainment for the Central Africans. Mac, for example, got off on the wrong foot when he was new to his post, and was being introduced to the *Chef de Village* (Village Chief). He courteously inquired about the health of the chef's family but lost a bit of traction when he asked about the status of the chef's big rear end. When I was up in Alindao once helping Tom with a pond-side training session, he got some puzzled looks from the fish farmers when he advised them to put notebooks in their ponds. To their credit, these farmers simply nodded as if they were receiving sage counsel from Tom. I did not detect any snickering. They would wait for the evening fire to share the story with their families. Then there would have been considerable laughter. Peg certainly got the attention of her audience when she advised her class (in Sango) to coat the wood for their outhouse construction with used motor oil, to prevent the penises from eating it. I have no recollection of any misspoken words on my part.

Our first weeks in Africa remained just a series of pleasant daily adventures, so long as we were together. The five months of training was intended to prepare us for our solitary two-year assignments. But we were living day-to-day, enjoying each other's company, and never really thinking about what the future had in store for us. I guess it is called *denial*. My post was to be in Bangassou, a town as far east as the fisheries program went. We will visit Bangassou later, so for now it is enough to know that I did not find it to my satisfaction, and ended up happily settling in Mobaye, thanks, in large part, to Tom.

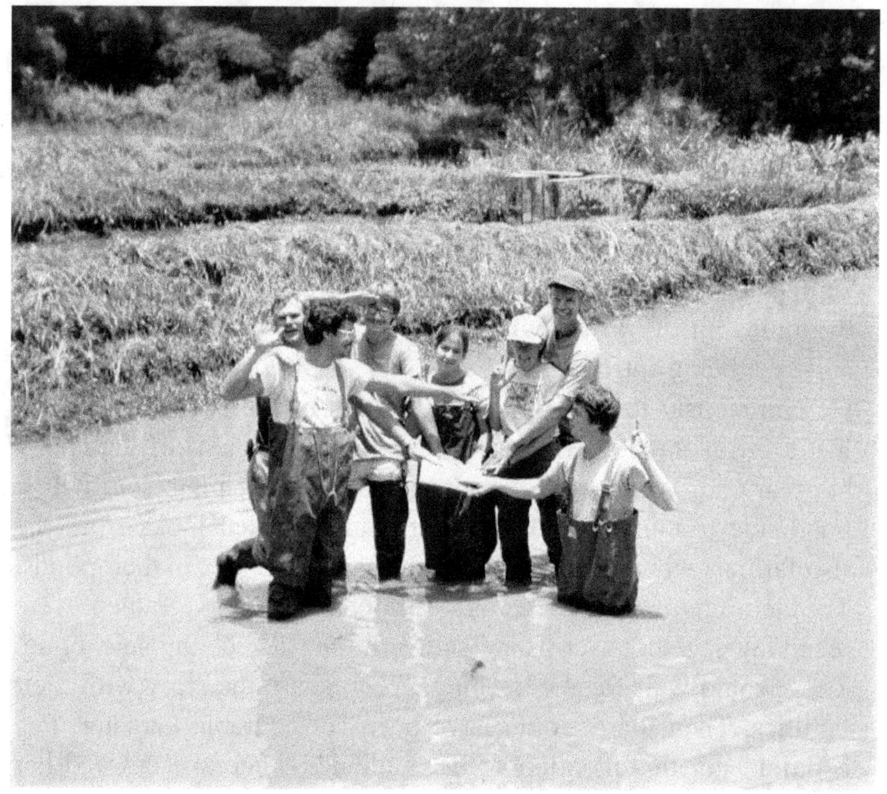

Swearing-in in M'Baiki. Left to right: me, Tom, Jerome and wife Pam (transfers), Rebecca, Mac and Pete

The CAR is about the size of Texas and is situated in the geographical center of the continent. While I was in Bangassou I was informed by a math volunteer that we were, in fact, at the geographical center. He had arrived at this conclusion by cutting the shape of the continent out of paper and balancing it on a pinhead. He said it balanced right on Bangassou. I thought this was pretty clever, especially for a math teacher.

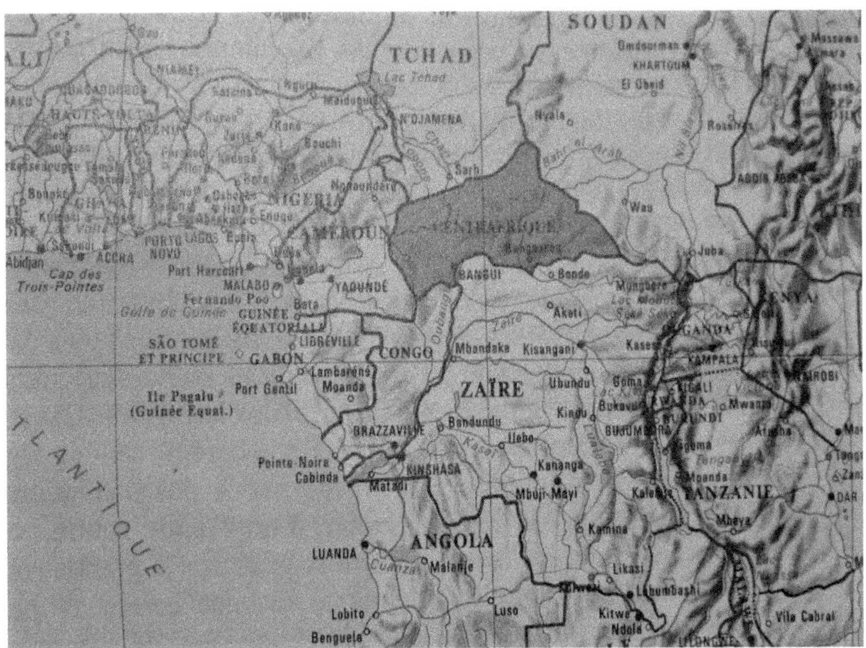

The CAR mostly borders on the south with what was then Zaire (now the Republic of Congo). The two countries were separated by the Oubangui and, further upstream, the Mbomou River. Bangassou, in the east, is on the Mbomou River, and Mobaye, in the south-central part of the country, is on the Oubangui River. Both Bangassou and Mobaye are prefectural capitals.

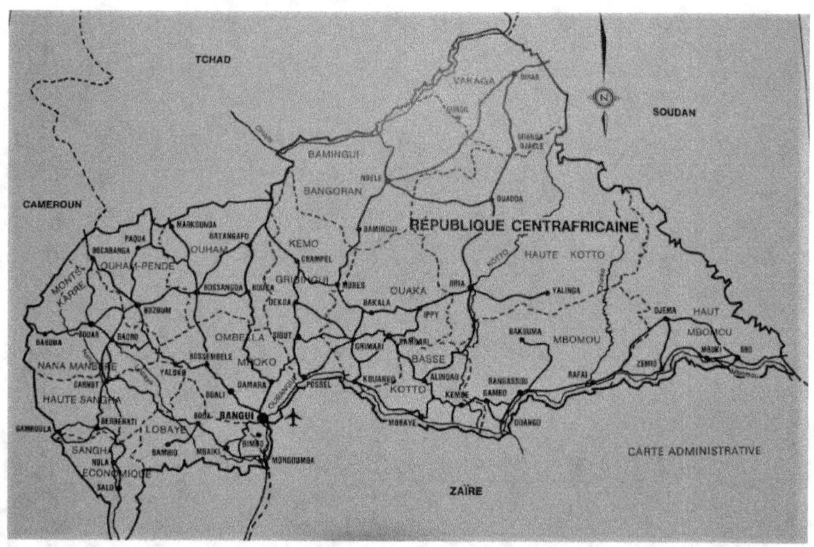

Mobaye, where we will be spending most of our time, is located about 500 kilometers east of Bangui, which is also situated on the Oubangui River. After whining long enough to my director, and with Tom's assistance, I moved to Mobaye in December of 1982. Tom had been assigned the entire Basse-Kotto prefecture, an area much too large for one person to cover.

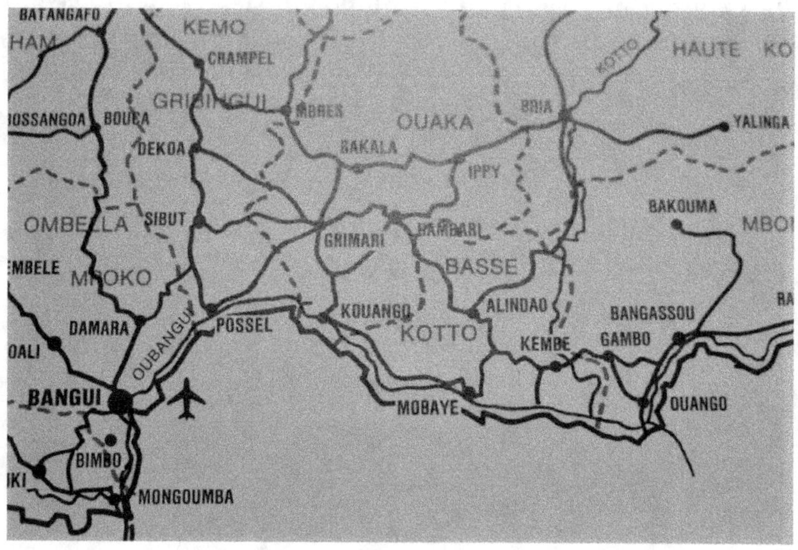

His argument to our director was that it made good sense to put two volunteers in the Basse-Kotto because it contained some of the best terrain for building ponds. Our director, after making a visit out to see the Basse-Kotto firsthand, bought the idea, and Tom and I could not have been happier. Tom took the northern half, stationed in a town called Alindao, and I took the southern half. Now the two boys from Minnesota were a mere 130 kilometers apart. The Basse-Kotto Boys had arrived.

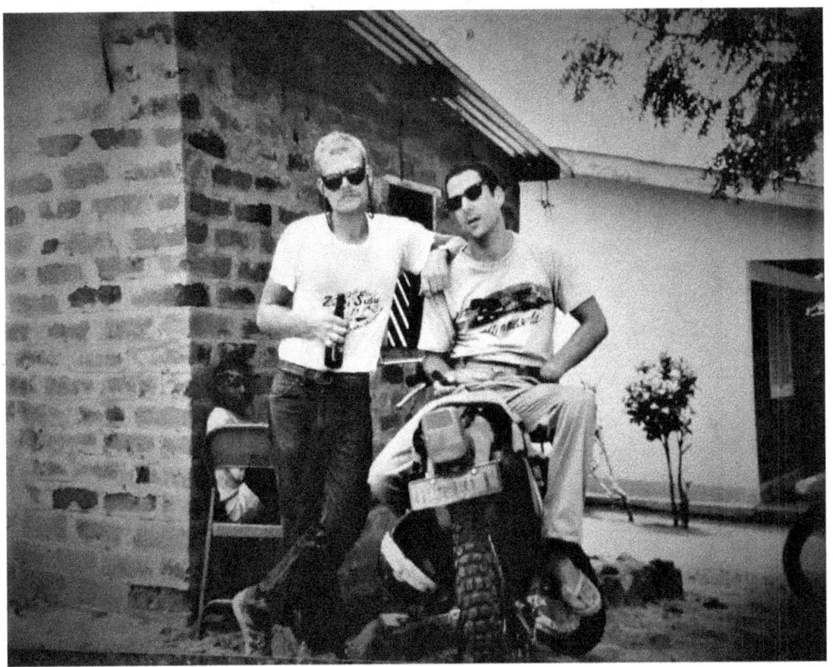

The Basse Kotto Boys in their glory days

Peg arrived in Mobaye in the fall of 1983, while I was stateside (more on that later). She worked in the school health program, where she initiated some cutting-edge disease-fighting procedures, such as handwashing. Peg lived in a mudbrick, dirt-floored, thatch-roofed house with a family in a neighborhood about a half mile from my house. She worked in the schools in the outlying villages, teaching basic sanitation and health practices to school children.

She traveled most days, when it was running, on a little blue moped.

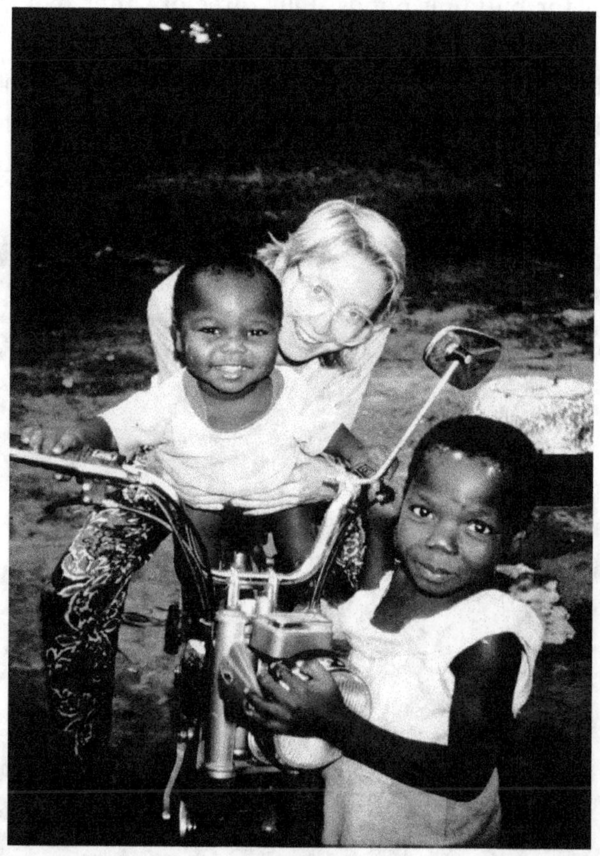

Peg and the neighbor kids

I, of course, was in the freshwater aquaculture program, teaching pond construction and fish farming techniques to farmers who were interested in raising tilapia for food and profit. Providing farmers with a source of income was, in fact, seen as more important for the health of a family than subsistence-level fish farming. This was a departure from the philosophy of the aquaculture program of the previous twenty years. The profit motive was pounded into us in Oklahoma, and we became dedicated to the capitalist mantra—which did not endear us to the more idealistic volunteers.

You may start to see that the fisheries volunteers had it pretty good. We were technically Peace Corps volunteers, but our project received its funding through the US Agency for International Development (USAID), making us the envy of the other, less well-funded volunteers. I lived in a mud-block house that, at one time, had a veneer of cement coating the bricks to dress it up a bit. Much of the coating had sloughed off, but enough remained to make it stand out as one of the more upscale residences in town. There was also a thin veneer of cement covering the dirt floor, which was mostly intact and made for much easier tidying up. The roof of the house was made of galvanized metal. This upgrade, more than anything else, made the place stand out as a symbol of affluence. Although much hotter than a thatched roof, a metal roof was made to last, and the gutter in front became the go-to place to gather water during the rainy season. My house was located right on *the strip*: the main road leading to the old colonial part of town, which was situated along the river.

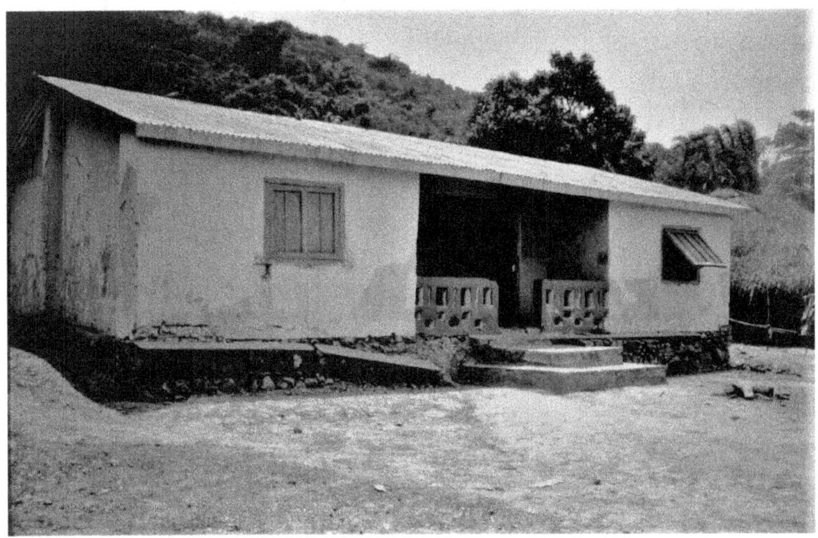

My house-front view

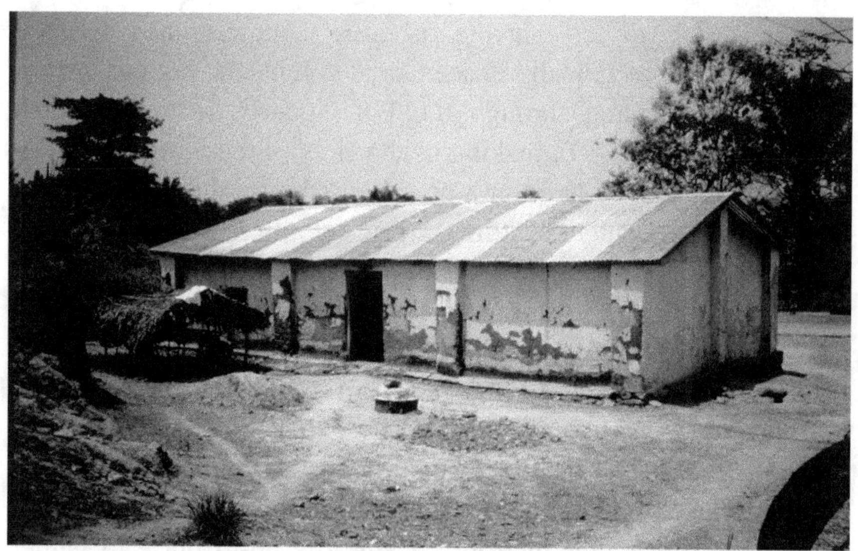

Rear view with a bit less curb appeal

I had, for daily use, a motorcycle (*moto*) and, for more than my fair share of the time, a four-wheel-drive diesel Toyota Land Cruiser pickup truck. Having a sleek 125 cc Suzuki also gave me an edge at getting a date with Peg, since our first date was a trip to the dirt airstrip to teach her how to drive a motorcycle. If the motorcycle wasn't enough, the truck was the real chick magnet.

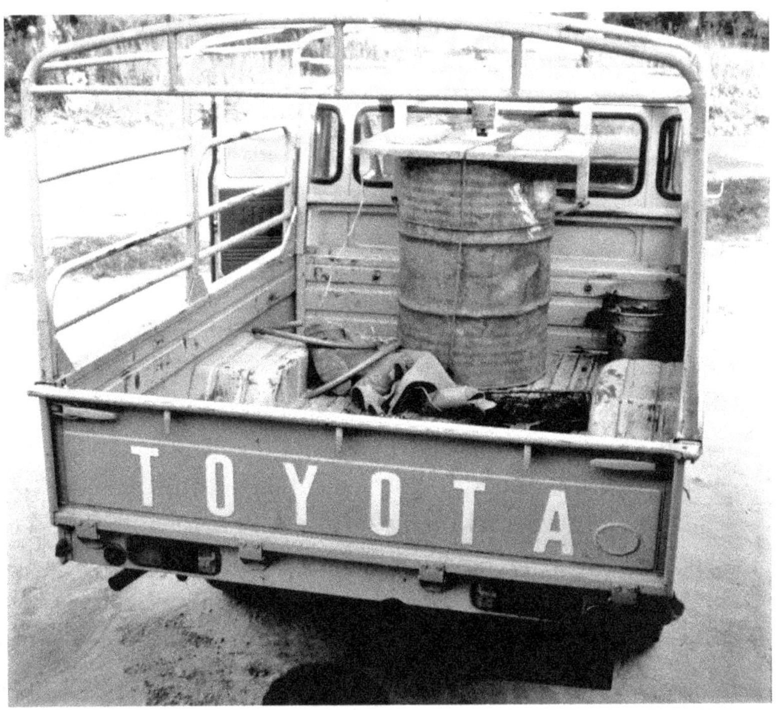

Fisheries truck-loaded with fingerlings for Oye´Carrefour

THE FOOD

ood in Mobaye was obtained daily from a morning market down by the river in the *Centre Ville* (town center). This was the main market, where cattle were slaughtered and freshly caught fish was available seasonally, along with a large assortment of fresh fruits and vegetables. Usually, it was the cook of the household who went to this market to procure the food for the main meal of the day, which was served at noon. The workday began at sunrise. Being just ten degrees north of the equator meant that sunrise was—at most—fifteen minutes on either side of 6 a.m., year-round. It was therefore up to my cook to shop at the morning market for my noon meal.

That statement may get some of you thinking that this guy was one of those self-important Americans who would exploit the poor and treat them like slave laborers; and that is exactly how I first viewed those who hired servants. I was much more comfortable fending for myself. Then it was explained to me by our director that hiring a servant was an expectation *and an obligation* for a volunteer, and not exploitation. Central Africans also saw it as an obligation. I was considered a wealthy person, so to not share my wealth was seen as selfish and downright greedy. It was a difficult concept to grasp at first, since I received only a living allowance, not a salary. It took a while to realize that the typical villager lived for an entire year on what I received in two weeks.

So, I hired Celestin, the cook who more-or less came with the house. I was an amazingly lame *patron*, which Celestin must have found puzzling. He was a fine man, husband, and father who, no doubt, entertained his family around the evening fires with tales about his pushover patron who did not know how to treat a servant like a servant. But after seeing how servants were treated by the wealthier Africans and the Lebanese expatriates who abused and beat them, I was okay with being a lightweight patron. Celestin may have had a gravy job compared to his counterparts, but he still worked hard, and he made amazing meals over a three-rock fire in my backyard

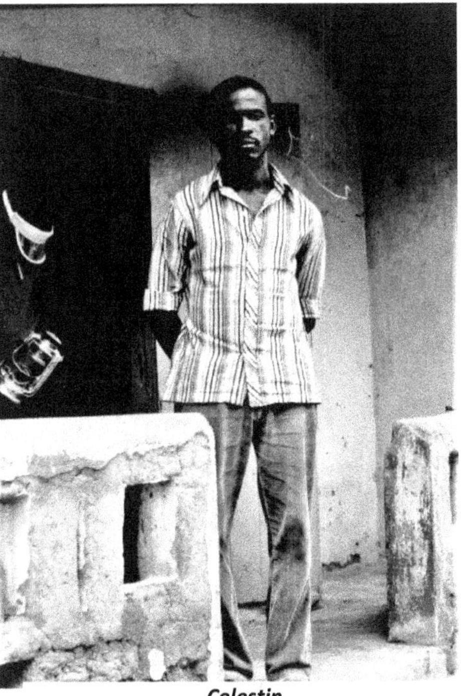

Celestin

Besides shopping and cooking, he carried my disgustingly dirty work clothes down to the river at least once a week and washed them. It may be trendy here now, but we had the authentic stone-washed blue jeans. During the rainy season, Celestin got off a bit easier because the gutter on the front of my house became the primary domestic water supply. Barring a rainstorm, I had a twenty-foot-deep dug well in the backyard, which was shared with the neighbors to supplement the water supply. The dry season, however, was another story. It lived up to its name, and we could go weeks without precipitation. In the dry, oppressive heat, everything turned brown and my well went dry. Celestin was then forced to walk a mile to a spring-fed stream every day to collect water in a twenty-liter marmite (large aluminum pot). Anyone who had carried forty pounds of water on top of their head for a mile every day for six months had, in my opinion, earned their two dollars for the day.

With just five gallons of water to get through the day, I quickly learned to use it frugally. We will discuss wastefulness later, but for now it is enough to mention that scarcity breeds frugality. A typical shower used about two gallons of water, which was entirely adequate. I was sometimes a bit of a resource hog, though, and warmed the water in a metal bucket over the fire before metering it out over myself with a metal coffee cup.

Along with the winter dry season came the hot, dry days. It was not unusual for my thermometer to read 100 degrees, with occasional spurts up to 110. Most of the villages with fishponds, or pond construction sites, were ten to twenty kilometers north or west of Mobaye, so I would generally arrive there within an hour after sunrise, and the workday was over promptly at noon. This most practical of traditions was necessary due to the extreme heat of the noonday sun. As it approached noon, I would begin to check my watch and plan my escape. The villagers were perfectly willing to work right up to the noon knock-off time since they were already home. They only had to wander over to the *paillote* (a thatch-roofed pavilion) to share a calabash of cool palm wine and enjoy a hot meal prepared by their spouse. I, on the other hand, had to drive my moto at unsafe speeds, dodging chickens along treacherous roads, to make it to Henri's boutique on the north side of Mobaye.

After several hours of work in the desiccating heat, I would begin to crave a bottle of Henri's ice-cold Coca-Cola. By 11:30, it became an obsession to get to that little store before it closed promptly at noon. Looking back, it is funny that the only time in my life that I wore a wristwatch was while I was working in a place in the world where time should have had little relevance. The fish farmers and agents I worked with, however, were sticklers for punctuality. If I said I would be there at 6:30, they would be very disappointed in me if I was late for any reason. So, I wore a watch to keep them happy and so I could get to Henri's boutique before he closed. Henri kept his pop and beer in a kerosene-powered freezer, which did not work quite well enough to freeze anything, but kept the beverages hovering just above freezing. The beer brewery in Bangui, called Mocaf, was also the distributor for Coca-Cola and Fanta orange soda. The Coke was bottled in roughly ten-ounce, heavy, old-style green-tinted bottles so they would survive the journey in wooden cases stacked in open transport trucks, as they rattled over the rough roads. Central Africans were not fond of cold beverages, but Henri knew what his wealthier customers wanted, and so he served up the coldest drinks in town. He was a shrewd businessman, but Henri would stay open past noon for no one. I would race into his shop, covered in red dust, and plop my change on the counter. Looking at his watch, he would then serve me my ice-cold bottle of Coca-Cola. Then he would stand back, fold his arms, and watch the show. I was the only customer who could consume such a numbingly cold liquid in less than ten seconds.

I could not make it to Henri's store every day, of course. I had been fortunate enough to have procured a kerosene-powered refrigerator from a terminating volunteer, in a town called Kembé, about one hundred kilometers away. Once again, having a truck at my disposal proved to be handy. A refrigerator was an almost unheard-of extravagance, even for Peace Corps volunteers. They were expensive to purchase, difficult to transport (without a truck), temperamental to maintain, and rather expensive to operate. But the alternative was to have warm beer, so I really saw no choice in the matter. Besides having cold beer, coming home at noon to a bottle of ice-cold water was almost as good as Henri's Coca-Cola. Warm, iodized water was just not something worth rushing home for. Before chugging the water, I would pour a good palmful of salt into my hand and eat it. It's funny how we are so sodium-phobic here in America, but in the CAR, after six hours in the tropical sun, I craved salt as much as I craved water. Once my thirst was quenched, the other thing I had visions of while riding home was one of Celestin's noon meals.

Every morning, before I headed out to the villages, I would give Celestin some cash and entrust him with the task of shopping for the noonday meal. I usually left the menu planning up to him, since it was generally based on what was plentiful that day. If there were fresh fish available at a reasonable price, the meal would usually include fish, which was only available fresh during the dry season. The Oubangui River swelled to the top of its banks during the rainy season and had dangerous currents that made fishing from a *pirogue* (a dug-out canoe) all but impossible.

Only smoked and dried fish were available during the rainy season. This preservation technique is not to be confused with the flavorful brined and smoked fish we are accustomed to. These were large chunks of fish that had been caught in nets at the end of the dry season and hung over a smoldering fire to partially dehydrate and encrust them in particulates from the smoke. No salt was used in this process, and the preservation method was inadequate, at best. It had an aroma of decomposition that I found unappetizing, and the chunks containing maggots were even less tempting. I instructed Celestin to stick with the fresh fish. Being relatively expensive, even for a high roller like me, I seldom ate whole fish unless they were small ones. Usually, I ate a small amount of fish served in a sauce, but when they were plentiful and reasonably priced, Celestin would create a masterpiece. He would scale and clean (but not head) the fish, cut diagonal slits through the skin, make a paste of palm oil, minced garlic, onion, and salt, and baste the fish with it as it roasted over hot coals. He then served the golden-brown fish on a bed of seasoned rice.

Shoppers went to the morning market for fresh beef. By fresh, I mean the cattle were herded past my house early in the morning on the way to the market and were herded back—minus one member—in the early afternoon. The cattle, dark brown, long-horned, skeletal creatures with long droopy ears, belonged to nomadic cattle herders called the Mbororo. The entire herd was brought to the market, where all but one was kept inside of a wooden-poled corral. The unfortunate creature selected for slaughter was prodded and pulled up onto a concrete-floored, three-sided structure that reminded me of a stage. This was where the whole production was performed for the shoppers. I watched the process one time, and that was enough for me. As the meat and highly prized entrails were hacked from the carcass, customers would line up to place their orders, which were then packaged in banana leaves. The entire operation, from start to cleanup, with a few buckets of water from the river, took only a couple of hours. Sanitation standards were not what we are accustomed to here in the States. Probably the most effective sanitizing agent was the sizzling tropical sun, but it had little effect on the fly population.

This scene played out every week in the market, and anyone who could afford it would buy a portion of the animal to have some animal protein in their sauce. I knew of no one, however, who would buy a steak or a roast and eat a large chunk of it, as we do in America. For one thing, it was physically impossible to chew this meat if it was cut thicker than a quarter inch. It was also too expensive for most folks to purchase large quantities. The meat was sometimes thinly sliced, seasoned, skewered, grilled over coals, and sold as market food. The more reputable of these booths were quite popular. Although their diet was based mostly on manioc, peanuts, vegetables, and fruits, Central Africans loved to have some meat included in their sauces. The first choice would have been wild game, and I suspect this goes back through the mists of time, to when a successful hunt meant a time of plenty. The game was virtually gone from where I lived, but the desire for meat to boost the everyday stew pot was still strong in the CAR. It was not really possible for the average person to get too much meat. It was simply too expensive to buy, too scarce to hunt, and too capital- and labor-intensive to raise animals for food. Pigs, sheep, goats, and chickens were raised, but they were always free-range creatures, and how villagers knew who owned what was beyond me. Central Africans craved animal protein as much as I craved salt.

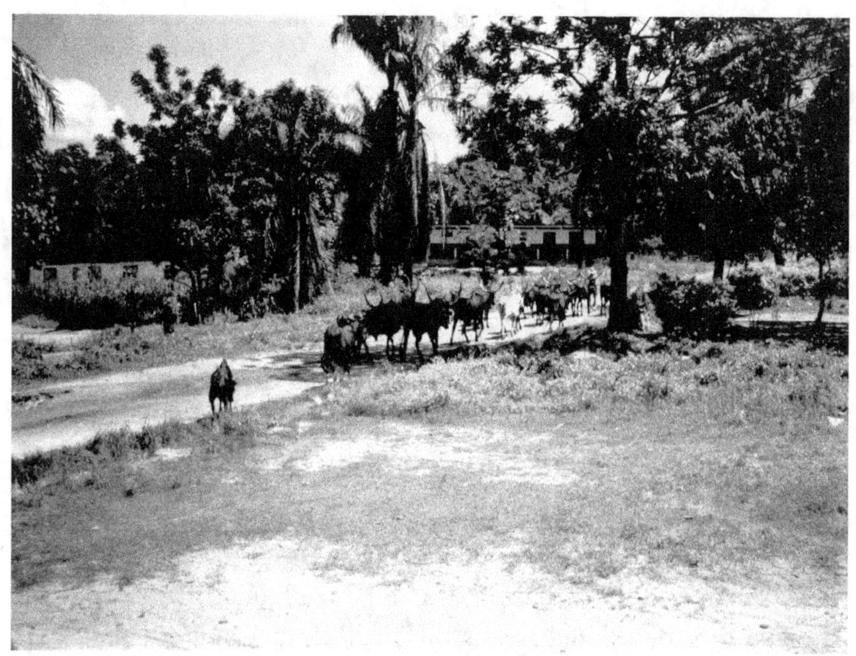

The cattle herd-minus one member-leaving the morning market

The first rains of the season signaled the swarming of termites, which was a cause for celebration. There was a frenzy of activity as both kids and adults scampered about, cramming every termite they could catch into their mouths. When they had their fill, some of the delectable insects were saved to be fried up in palm oil and seasoned with salt, for their version of fireside popcorn in the evenings.

When the dry season desiccated the savanna, it was time for a rat roundup. This meant that it was time to strategically burn the grasslands to flush out the resident rodents. Hunting these gerbil-like creatures reminded me a bit of deer opener in Minnesota. The rat chasers and rat catchers chattered excitedly as the rodents ran ahead of the flames, being chased down by stick- wielding rat hunters reveling in this short-lived bonanza of free animal protein. It amazed me that these folks were willing to expend so much energy during the hottest time of the year in pursuit of a few ounces of animal flesh. But such was their desire to enjoy a few skewers of roasted rats during this short-lived time of relative plenty.

After I left the CAR and returned home to Minnesota, Peggy still had a year remaining in her service. In one of the letters I sent to her in the fall of 1984, I included several pictures of me posing with harvested grouse, ducks, and deer. When Peg shared these photos with her Central African friends, she was strongly advised to marry me because I was obviously a great hunter. Being a good hunter meant being a good provider, and there was no higher value to be placed on a husband.

It was mainly the women who planted and harvested crops and gathered the greens for the daily meal. If the husband was not bringing home game, he was likely to be found sitting in the shade, drinking palm wine, and awaiting dinner. Any wild creature that was seen was killed with the ever-ready machete, unless it was unsafe to do so without being bitten. Birds or tree-dwelling monkeys were killed using homemade shotguns fashioned out of iron water pipe for the barrels and hand-carved stocks. Only the military could possess firearms, but the villagers found a loophole and somehow got away with owning these homemade shotguns for hunting. These firearms appeared to me to be just as lethal for the hunters as for the hunted. Unfortunate little monkeys were displayed along the roadside for sale, after a slit was made through their necks, and the tail was pulled through the slit to create a handy hanger for displaying their game from a forked stick stuck in the ground. After a day or two hanging in the sun, the price would be reduced for quick sale.

Central Africans are deathly afraid of snakes. I don't know what possessed Tom to do it, but he thought it would be fun to bring a realistic-looking rubber snake with him to the CAR. During one of our first meetings with the Central African language teachers, Tom unexpectedly lobbed this snake onto the lap of one of them. I have never heard such a high-pitched scream come from a male, as he levitated and threw the snake across the room. Africans love slapstick humor and practical jokes, but this was way over the top. It took a long time to quiet the teachers, who were all cowering in a corner of the room. None of them were laughing. Even after they calmed down and were assured that the snake was, indeed, made from rubber (and that Tom should be allowed to live) none of these grown men could get themselves to touch the fake snake.

In their defense, there was good reason to fear snakes; a bite from a poisonous one meant certain death. I thought of this many times as I waded through streambeds, occasionally grasping tree limbs to keep my balance, knowing that a perfectly camouflaged green mamba could be coiled around any of those limbs. Our advice, if we were to be bitten by a mamba, was to enjoy (as much as possible) the ten minutes remaining in our lives. Snakes were sometimes caught in the fishponds during a harvest, causing a frenzy of whooping and machete wielding as the unfortunate creature was hacked to pieces. Pythons are not poisonous, but they are still snakes. Their other downfall is that they are quite tasty. Although they were rare—since any python seen was automatically a dead python—I did eat python on two occasions, and it really was delicious.

I also dined on termites, smoked zebra and elephant smuggled in from Zaire, and caterpillars. These were huge, green, smooth-skinned caterpillars that lived in the rain forests around M'Baiki. After they were fried in palm oil and seasoned with salt and hot red pepper, they tasted surprisingly like breakfast sausages (except for the head, which had a rather unappetizing crunch to it). Trying these exotic foods was necessary to avoid offending my hosts and, perhaps more importantly, to shock the folks back home. Even if I had only tried these foods a time or two, when asked what I ate in Africa, I could honestly say, "Oh, termites, monkeys, pythons, zebra, elephant, and caterpillars. You know, the usual stuff." I drew the line at what Tom and I saw being vended at a market in Gabon, though. While perusing the market, we were shocked to see a woman carrying the entire arm of a great ape. It saddened us to see the dismembered bodies of an endangered primate for sale as food.

We knew a few Central African teachers who had been awarded the rare opportunity to travel to the United States to further their studies. Joseph, a high school teacher in Mobaye, was one of those who had been to America. When asked what most impressed him about the States, he did not hesitate in his response. "Kentucky Fried Chicken," he said. Chickens in the CAR were like little feathered marathon runners, with skin that was tightly stretched over a scrawny skeleton, and a thin covering of well-conditioned muscle in between. This is the type of chicken Joseph had grown up believing was a once- or twice-a-year luxury food. So, to be presented with a piece of breast meat that weighed more than a whole CAR chicken, a piece of meat permeated with succulent juices and coated with an extra-crunchy breading containing eleven herbs and spices, well, it was almost too much for the guy.

The sauces in the CAR were typically based on *pate d'arachide*, or peanut butter. Peanuts were planted, grown, harvested, and processed by hand, usually by the women. I will point out here that there were no fungicides, pesticides, or fertilizers used on crops or even available to farmers. They may not have been certified, but they were certainly organic. Fields were tilled and cultivated by hand, usually by women bent over short-handled, hand-forged hoes, for hours on end. Many of the women would perform these tasks with newborn infants strapped snugly to their backs. These women also hand-planted and harvested the crops, irrigated them with water carried on their heads from nearby streams, and carried the harvest back to the village for processing, which was also their job. Hand-harvested peanuts were shelled, roasted in a kettle over the fire, and then pounded into a paste in a wooden mortar and pestle. The mortar and pestle, next to the cooking pot, was the most essential piece of food preparation equipment that the family owned. Hewn from a solid log, a mortar could be passed on for generations. Peanut butter was sold in the markets wrapped in a banana leaf. It was intended for use in sauces, but us zany Americans actually ate the stuff as is, or on bread or bananas. Some enterprising women saw a business opportunity and added salt and sugar to make it taste more like the peanut butter we were accustomed to. What we were not accustomed to, however, was the parasite load that generally accompanied the peanut butter. It was not an issue when it was cooked in a sauce, but we were eating it straight out of the mortar, which had not been sanitized between uses (or even between generations).

Onion and garlic were, thankfully, plentiful, and relatively inexpensive to purchase, so they were usually part of the sauce, first sautéed in red palm oil. Palm oil was also locally produced by the women in the villages. The ripe palm fruits were first harvested by climbing the palm, which was the man's job, or by gathering fallen fruits from under the palm. The fruits were first boiled to soften them, and then dumped into the mortar and pounded with the pestle into a fibrous mash. This mash was then squeezed by hand into a pot, which was heated over the fire to evaporate the water, leaving behind the deep orange-red semisolid oil. This unrefined oil contained both saturated and unsaturated fats, along with some of the remaining fiber. It was also packed with carotenoids and members of the vitamin E family of antioxidants. In short, it was cooking oil that was also a wholesome food. After returning to the States I tried, in vain, to find red palm oil. I could only find the white, highly refined palm oil, with all the good stuff removed. Now, thirty-some years later, thanks to online global shopping, we did find some red palm oil, although it came from plantations in Indonesia and lacked the flavor and aroma of freshly pressed palm oil.

A green of some sort was usually added to the sauce. Many spinach-type plants grew wild. Some were herbaceous and others were vines that grew everywhere year-round. Gathering a pile of greens was not a problem if you knew what to look for. I entrusted Celestin with the greens collection. Sometimes, manioc leaves were added. A leaf called *koko*, which was stacked and chopped into thin strands, was popular. To me, it tasted like a pile of lawn clippings dumped into an otherwise perfectly good sauce. It was Tom's favorite meal, but I visited him anyway. For a special occasion, a chicken would be sacrificed and added to the sauce. Next, hot red pepper (by *hot* I mean the thinking-you-might-die kind of hot) was always added to the sauce. Once it was ready, a large *boule* (ball) of a grey, rubbery mass fondly known as *gozo* was inevitably served with the sauce.

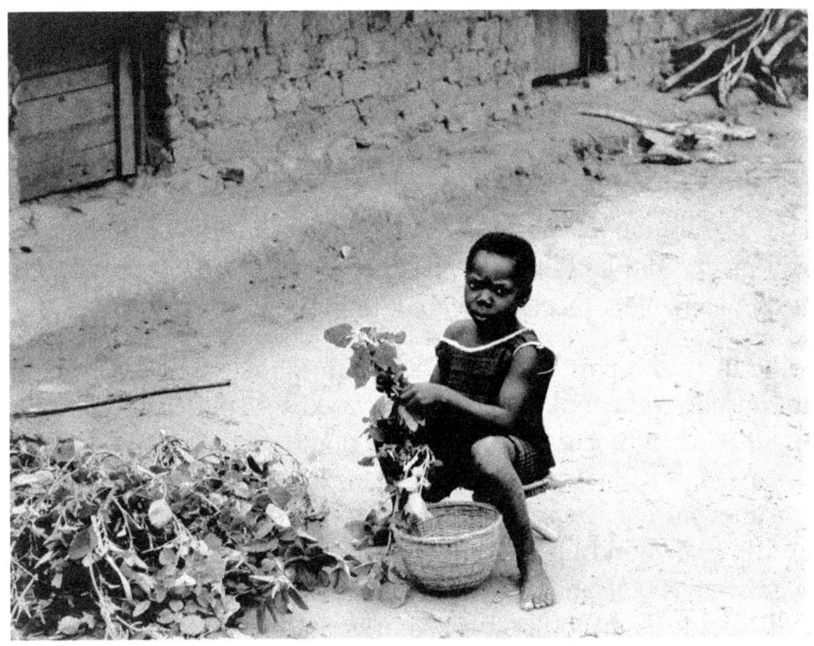

Preparing the greens- a big pile of them

Gozo was made from manioc, or *cassava* as it is called in its native South America, and most meals centered around it. Manioc was so firmly entrenched in the culture that I was amazed to learn that it is not native to Africa. I guess it's a bit like tomatoes and Italian cuisine. It is hard to believe that tomatoes were unknown in Europe until the 1500s. Prior to the introduction of manioc, plantains (which are native to Indonesia but had arrived in Africa well before manioc) had been the starch of choice for Central Africans, along with yams. But they loved their manioc, if not for its flavor (there really was none) then for its caloric density and its ability to add bulk to an otherwise sparse meal. Manioc filled people up and added calories in the form of complex carbohydrates. It was an inexpensive meal extender. It was not easy to produce, however. In fact, it was such a terribly labor-intensive process that I found it puzzling that they bothered with it—especially considering the taste, odor, and texture of the end product.

The first step in the creation of gozo was to harvest the tubers of the spindly, woody, kind of homely, palmate-leaved shrub. The roots were then peeled and placed in a small stream for a few days to leach out the cyanide compounds that naturally occur in manioc roots. Hearing the word *cyanide*, one might think that this is something best left alone. But no, they persist, and carry the waterlogged tubers back to the village, where they are broken into small pieces and laid out on an old, rusty sheet of steel roofing, or onto a clean-swept piece of ground, to ferment and dry.

Riding my moto past a batch of fermenting manioc, I would be hit with an odor that took some getting used to—but in fact, I never did get used to it. The closest thing I could compare that aroma to was my high school gym locker when it was opened for the first time after spring break. The dried, fermented chunks of manioc were then gathered up and bagged into burlap sacks to be sold in the local market. Enough of the chunks would be held back for the family and brought to the trusty mortar and pestle to be pulverized into manioc flour. To prepare a boule for the meal, hot water would be stirred into the flour until it formed the grey, gym-sock-smelling, Silly-Putty-textured substance that was adoringly dipped into the flavorful sauces

FRESH FRUITS GALORE

The quality, quantity, and variety of fresh fruits was amazing—especially to a kid from Minnesota. I had never even heard of a papaya, for example, before coming to the CAR. I quickly learned that a ripe papaya, sliced lengthwise with the seeds scooped out and squirted with lime juice, was heavenly. It was reminiscent of the cantaloupe I was accustomed to but had an exotic flavor and texture that was new to me.

Then there were pineapples. I had seen the commercials on TV showing the whole pineapple being sucked into a can in Hawaii. My only experience with pineapple was in finding chunks of canned pineapple entombed in a Jell-O salad. I had never seen an actual pineapple fruit or the plant that it comes from. I was intrigued to learn that they are a spiny shrub and the fruit grows up from the center of it, upside down from my perspective. But boy, were they good. I had my first golden, totally ripe, aromatic pineapple when I was a lonely soul at my first post in Bangassou. They were so good that I kind of went on a pineapple-eating binge. At first, I could not understand why I had to visit the cabinet (outhouse of sorts) so frequently during the night, until one evening when I hung my prized pineapple from my fish scale and saw that it weighed in at over seven pounds. Since they are mostly water, it turns out I had been consuming close to a gallon before turning in for the night. I was relieved to find out that I did not have some strange tropical disease (yet). I did, however, start eating pineapples in moderation, and earlier in the evening (which was a bit hard to do since I went to bed about 7 p.m.).

Having mentioned my cabinet, I will elaborate on them here. The cabinet at the house in Mobaye was classy. The pit was quite deep, and it was a true outhouse, complete with walls, a thatched roof, and a door (but no seat). The one in Bangassou, on the other hand, consisted of a shallow pit enclosed by a rickety curtain of woven palm fronds. It was soon apparent that the user of this cabinet became much too intimate with the contents of the shallow hole that became a bit less deep every day. I was soon forced to hire a local latrine expert to remedy this situation. His solution was to, rather than dig a new hole, build up the ground around the existing hole. Unfortunately, he did not see the need to correspondingly increase the height of the palm frond curtain. So, in the mornings, I would find myself perched on top of what looked like a pitcher's mound, the upper two-thirds of my body visible over the top of the curtain, as a stream of market goers waved from the road.

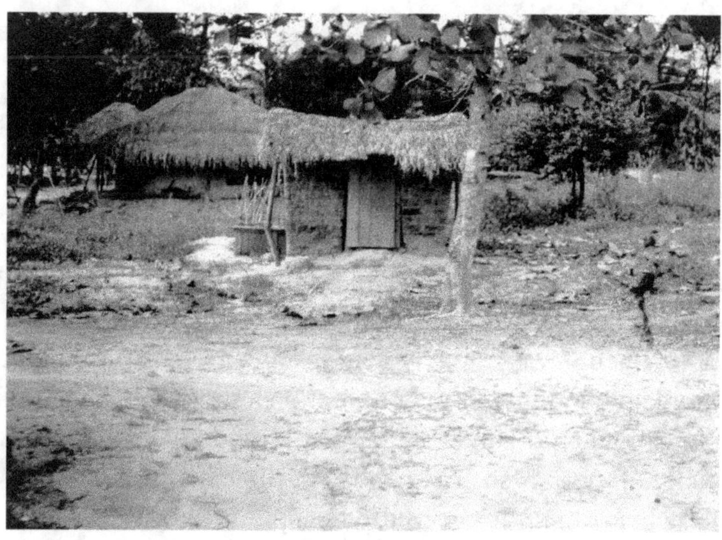

The Mobaye cabinet was classy

Now back to fruit. Citrus fruits were abundant during the rainy season, and I was surprised to learn that oranges in Africa, even when fully ripe, were green. But they were orange and juicy on the inside and were usually consumed as an all-natural juice box. The outer skin would be peeled off with the ever-present machete, leaving the white pithy layer intact. The top was then cut off and the fruit was squeezed while the juice was drunk through the opening. There were discarded biodegradable juice boxes strewn everywhere when oranges were dropping from the trees and were free for the taking. The free-range pigs could not have been happier. Limes, lemons, and grapefruit were also seasonally cheap and plentiful. Grapefruit, I noted, tasted no better over there than it does here. I guess absolute freshness has its limits. Limes accompanied the previously mentioned papayas and were paired with another fruit that was a new discovery for me: the avocado.

Mangoes were yet another previously unknown fruit for me. We need to remember that this was the early 1980s, and I was from Minnesota. Although these fruits are available in Minnesota supermarkets nowadays, growing up, the only tropical fruits I ever saw were bananas and citrus. Although I see tropical fruits now in supermarkets here in Bemidji, I am seldom tempted to purchase them (except for plantains, but we'll talk about that later). Having experienced absolutely-fresh tropical fruits, these poor geriatric fruits look worn out from way too much traveling. Getting back to mangoes, they must be completely ripe to be properly peeled and eaten. Consuming a ripe mango is an outdoor activity. To peel a mango, first make four shallow slices from end to end, and then peel away each skin segment to reveal the juicy, yellow flesh. I thought that mangoes tasted somewhat like peaches, but with an exotic, tropical flavor to them. The mangoes in Mobaye were of a generic variety, and I thought they all tasted about the same until Tom and I tasted a variety grown in Cameroon. These mangoes tasted like a cross between bananas and bubble gum. They were like eating candy, and the pit in the center was smaller and much less fibrous than the Mobaye variety, which was so fibrous that eating too close to the pit annoyingly embedded the fibers between my teeth.

When other fruit trees had shut down their production until the rains returned, the mighty mango trees with their deep roots took center stage as the saviors of the dry season. They became so plentiful that the market vendors gave up trying to sell them. The fruit was free for the taking by anyone who walked under the massive trees that lined and shaded the roads. These relics of past French colonialism remained from the era when France had commandeered much of Equatorial Africa in pursuit of the natural resources that were not found in abundance within their own borders. In Mobaye, the mango-tree-lined roads, along with the shells of the former colonial structures along the river, were the only physical evidence remaining from this colonial period. The Central African government still used many of these buildings, where *functionaires* (government officials) sat at old wooden desks in their sad, rather pathetic attempt to model themselves after the French system of prefectural governance.

Seeing bananas growing for the first time was another thrill for me. Most of the bananas eaten by Central Africans were the small ones, and the red variety, having a hint of strawberry flavor, was my favorite. Because they were small, thin-skinned, fragile, and quick to over-ripen, it is understandable that these are not the varieties to be grown in Central America and shipped to Minnesota. The bananas that we are accustomed to eating in Minnesota are the ones that the Central Africans would toss to the pigs. Plantains, the larger, starchier cousin of the banana, along with yams, were the carbohydrate staples prior to the introduction of manioc. Both have now taken a backseat to gozo, but they still have a good presence in the markets. Yams the size of a human leg—some complete with appendages that looked strikingly like human toes—had deeply wrinkled skin that made them difficult to peel. I was never crazy about them. Plantains, on the other hand, were wonderfully sweet and soft when they were fully ripe.

Plantains may be purchased here in northern Minnesota, and we buy them to satisfy our occasional cravings for our favorite African meal, but they have a lot of miles on them and were picked when they were still hard and green. When they do eventually ripen, the skin tends to adhere to the flesh, which is somewhat astringent, even when ripe. Not so with freshly harvested, completely ripe plantains. I preferred them raw to bananas, which were almost too much like eating candy. Plantains had substance, and the starches, which were not fully converted to sugars, gave them an appealing, smooth texture. Plantains starred in what was to become my all-time favorite meal, one that I am certain Celestin got tired of preparing so frequently, which he called simply *sauce tomate*. It was a peanut butter sauce packed with chopped tomatoes, spinach, onion, garlic, palm oil, and some hot pepper, served over ripe plantains that had been fried in palm oil. Peg and I love it, and I will share the recipe with you at the end as a reward for finishing this book.

THE AFTERNOON MARKET

As we discussed, there was the main morning market down along the river in Centre Ville. But at a crossroads on the north end of town, and a short walk from my house, was the *post-sieste* (after the nap) market. The afternoon market, like the morning market, was bordered by three-sided permanent booths that were occupied by the *Arabs*, a generic term for anyone of the Muslim faith and wearing a white robe. These merchants sold everything from canned goods, such as sardines and tomato paste, to essentials like toothpaste, cloth, lanterns, flashlights, batteries, toilet tissue, candles, and matches. Most of these items, even back then, were made in China and were of amazingly poor quality. I got a kick out of the toilet paper, which when unwrapped, revealed a center tube about twice the diameter of what we are accustomed to. The thin veneer of paper around the huge core made this purchase less of a bargain, and we simply went back to the *Newsweek International* magazines that all Peace Corps volunteers received. Fortunately, this edition was printed on newsprint. Glossy paper, for obvious reasons, had no place in the cabinet except as reading material.

The afternoon market was more of a casual affair and social event. It was a place where we went to pick up breakfast food and something to accompany the leftover noon meal for supper. This was a fun market, and I walked to it most afternoons. It took some planning though, since it was easy to dally and be caught, literally, in the dark. The market began at about 4 p.m., following the very sensible practice of taking a nap after the noon meal. On the shortest day of the year (December 21), the sun would set at 5:45 p.m. On the longest day (June 21), it would set at 6:15 p.m. The sun, near the equator, pops straight up in the morning and dives straight down at night, so there is no twilight. Like throwing a switch, it is light one minute and pitch dark (if there is no moon) the next. We usually had enough forethought to stick a flashlight in a shopping basket, but I recall a few instances of stumbling home by the unreliable light from an entire box of matches.

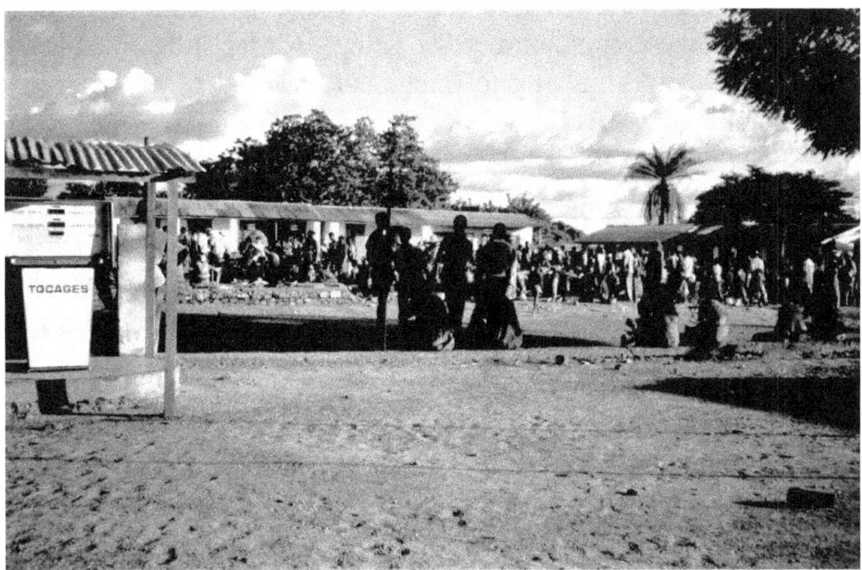

The afternoon market-seen from Henri's boutique

BREAD

I had a brass, single-burner kerosene stove that I had bought in Bangui before moving to Bangassou, and it was my savior. I did not have a cook in Bangassou and would prepare my evening meals on this little stove. I had not yet discovered the world of arriving home to a delicious hot meal at noon, so I limped along, snacking at noon and preparing my hot meal after dark (6 p.m.). A favorite dish of mine in Bangassou, besides pineapple, was sweet potato wedges fried in palm oil. I had discovered the red-skinned tubers in the market, and I would peel them, cut them into wedges, and then fry them in a good amount of palm oil until they were golden on the outside and tender on the inside. Served with salt and a bit of hot pepper, this was standard fare, accompanied by a can of sardines.

When I got to Mobaye, and had Celestin to prepare excellent noon meals, I used this stove to heat up the leftovers for supper. Some fresh fruit and bread from the afternoon market would usually accompany the leftovers. Yes, bread was usually available at the afternoon market and, being an American, I usually had to have bread with my meal. Wheat flour was one of those food items sometimes sold in the local shops. It was also one of those food items that really had no business being in Equatorial Africa, or at least not outside of the capital. Central Africans could take it or leave it. They had their gozo. But the French influence was still strong, and we Americans, as well as the expatriate population, loved bread. Beside baguettes, the other French-influenced dough product was the *beignet,* a deep-fried ball of sweet dough that tasted much like a doughnut. The beignet ladies were popular in markets closer to Bangui, where flour was fresher and more consistently available. But they were also made at the markets in Mobaye when there was flour in town.

The wheat flour that made its way to Mobaye was likely grown, milled, and bagged in France, and then shipped to a port in Cameroon. It then would have been transported overland in trucks to Bangui, and eventually distributed to the remote towns like Mobaye. Along the way, our flour became the home to countless flour beetles that lived out their lives, dining and excreting, in the bags of flour. Before we used it, all flour had to be sifted to screen out the bugs, but the aroma and flavor of flour beetle metabolic by-products lingered following their eviction. Some flour was less old than other flour, so when a supply of not-quite-so-old flour arrived, it was big news for those of us who were fond of bread. When it was available, there were enterprising bakers who made baguettes in mud-brick wood-fired outdoor ovens, and it really was quite good, considering the constraints they were under to effectively control the process. When flour was not readily available, however, some unscrupulous bakers would sneak in some manioc flour, resulting in a grey, dense loaf that had the taste and aroma of gym socks combined with a hint of cockroach droppings. Manioc bread usually made its way out the back door for the neighbor's pig.

There was some tolerable canned margarine available at the shops in Mobaye, but there was one English brand, made from fish oil, that I purchased just one time. Leave it to the British to make margarine from fish oil. I mostly ate my bread with peanut butter or canned sardines. The fast food of the CAR was a baguette and a can of Moroccan sardines, which were available everywhere for about twenty-five cents a can. These were the three-fish-per-can sardines, not the smaller ones from Norway that I used to eat out in the duck blind with my grandpa. They were good nonetheless, especially when we were hungry, and were quite handy when traveling. It is amazing how good food tastes when a person is experiencing real hunger. The best use I found for the bread was for sopping up the oil in the can once the sardines were consumed. There was little thought about limiting calories when I was thirty-five pounds underweight.

MY YOU ARE WELL FATTENED

There was no more flattering compliment in the CAR than to inform someone that they were good and fat. *Bien engraissé* was the way to tell someone that you have noticed that they are enviably living the good life. Anyone who is sporting body fat is showing the world that they have the means to buy foods that are scarce, expensive, and out-of-reach for most folks—-primarily Western foods made from refined carbohydrates. I became the recipient of these compliments following my return to the CAR, after a four-month-long medical evacuation to the States midway through my service.

I was driving my moto along a narrow roadway (part of the Trans-African Highway) during the rainy season. The dense, eight-foot-tall elephant grass growing up to the edge of the road, made it feel like I was driving through a green tunnel. Without warning, a large, pregnant, black-and-white goat leapt from the grass and stood right in my path. I only had time to stand up on the foot pegs before crashing to the road, with the full impact of the crash concentrated on my right kneecap. I quickly stood up to assess the damage, and promptly fell back down, since the main tendons that operated my knee had been smeared on the road. Fortunately, the crash had occurred on the outskirts of a small village. But then, if I had not been near a village, I would not have encountered a goat in the first place. Some villagers ran to me, carried me to a stool in the shade of a mango tree, pushed my moto off the road, and brought me a pan of water. I retrieved a bar of soap from my backpack and made a feeble attempt at cleaning the packed red dust from deep inside of my knee joint. I knew I was in trouble, so I shared the delectable macaroons I had stowed in my backpack with the villagers as I contemplated how I would get back to Bangui. I had just left Bangui that morning and was returning to Mobaye, following treatment for a fungal infection in my right foot. I had just left the infirmary, and now it looked like I was headed back there. Eventually. Somehow.

My trusty Red Wing Irish Setter work boots were the envy of every Central African male. The fish farmers always elected me to pack the pond banks during construction, since I wore *les grande bottes*—the big boots. While these boots offered pretty good protection for my feet, they also were an ideal breeding ground for the fungi that chose to call the skin between my toes home.

I say the boots were *pretty good* protection because, about six months earlier, while riding my moto along a narrow footpath to access a pond site, I got my left big toe caught between the foot peg and a large laterite rock. This is not the recommended method of stopping the forward progress of a 200-pound machine. I ended up breaking my big toe, an event that, up until that time, was the most pain I had ever experienced. My toe resembled a small black balloon, and for a couple of days I could only lie in bed popping the Benadryl tablets in my first aid kit. Even the slightest breeze passing over my toe caused severe pain.

Tom and I had been corresponding with a few of the other Oklahoma trainees who were stationed in Gabon, and they had invited us to visit them. Gabon is situated right on the equator, on the Atlantic coast of Africa. Not wanting to mess up plans for this trip, I immobilized my toe with some creative bandaging, and set off for Alindao, shifting with my heel the whole way. Tom and I then continued to Bangui, where I had hoped to have my toe x-rayed at the hospital. When we arrived, the hospital was without electricity, so nothing was done about my toe, which was feeling significantly better by then anyway.

Tom and I had planned to take *trafic* (privately run mass transit) from Bangui to Gabon, since driving our motos out of the country was frowned upon by our director. Somehow, we heard a rumor that the French military sometimes offered rides on their transport planes to government representatives traveling on official business. Anything was worth a try to avoid rattling around packed into the backs of trucks with a ridiculous number of other travelers and their livestock. We were, after all, representatives of the United States; it was the *official business* part that was a bit of a stretch. So that evening in the transit house (Peace Corps flophouse), I sat down at the typewriter and combined my persuasive writing skills with my burgeoning French to compose a letter to the base commander. I wrote,

Dear Commander: As biologists representing the United States of America in the CAR, working to implement modern aquaculture techniques to provide vital protein and income to subsistence-level farmers, my colleague and I feel it would be beneficial for us to observe the pond construction and management techniques being practiced by our counterparts in Gabon. We respectfully ask for your assistance in providing us with transport to Libreville, from whence we may embark on this mission...

Unfortunately, I did not have a complete command of the French language, and I thought it rather rude that this important military figure sat, cigarette dangling from his lips, reading my letter while chortling. What he was reading sounded more like this: *Dear Commander: We two USA fish mans want go to Gabon to watch fish tubs. We demand you us take on airplane to Libreville to go do big work...* I got the feeling that he was on to us, but he also took pity on me as I stood there attired in my cleanest red-dust-stained T-shirt and blue jeans, my dress flip-flops revealing my bandaged big toe. Despite my terrible letter, he agreed to transport us to Libreville on a flight leaving the following morning. Tom and I arrived bright and early with our duffel bags and strapped ourselves into the jump seats lining the windowless transport plane. We sat, with our scruffy beards and threadbare clothing, shoulder to shoulder with big, muscular, camouflage-uniformed French soldiers. But it got us to Libreville. *Vive la France!*

It was about six months after the trip to Gabon and Cameroon that I developed the fungal infection between and on all the toes on my right foot. It was the kind of infection that the writers of textbooks about tropical diseases searched for to add photos of worst-case scenarios. I had been treating the infection myself by mashing aspirin tablets into petroleum jelly and smearing it on my foot. This brought some temporary relief but did nothing to persuade the fungi to vacate my skin. The infection grew to the point that the pain became the worst I had ever experienced up to that point. I knew I was not going to fix this myself. So, with the right foot this time carefully bandaged, I set off on my moto for Bangui for treatment. It turned out that I also had a nasty secondary streptococcus infection that required a course of antibiotics and a couple of days spent immersing my foot in Betadine.

Once cured, I was on my moto headed back to Mobaye. This brings us back under the mango tree, where I left you so long ago. I was still attempting to clean packed red dust from a silver-dollar-sized hole over my right kneecap when a large flatbed truck came by and the driver was flagged down. Some of the men lifted my moto up into the back of the loaded truck, and then lifted me up into the spacious cab, where I could sprawl across the wide seat. The driver took me back toward Bangui to a town called Sibut, where there was an American Baptist mission. The driver would accept no payment for his kind act, saying his payment would be for me to help someone else out of a jam someday. As I was to experience, time after time, folk are folk. No matter where we go in the world, ordinary people are basically good. My good fortune was not to end there, since an American physician happened to be visiting the mission at the time. I felt bad that he and the nurse assisting him had to spend their entire evening and much of the night cleaning me up and stitching me back together.

When I was reassembled, the doctor warned me that, because it was impossible to clean the wound completely, the risk of infection was high. The next morning, the good folks from the mission loaded me up on a lounge chair in the back of a full-sized Ford pickup truck and drove me back to the Peace Corps infirmary, the place I had just left the morning before. Despite a course of antibiotics, my knee doubled in size and began to resemble a football, complete with the stitching. The pain became the worst I had ever experienced—up to that point. When the stitches could no longer withstand the pressure, the wound reopened and the decision was made to medically evacuate me to Washington, D.C. for treatment.

Because my right leg was splinted and could not bend, I was given a first-class ticket; the spacious seating would allow me to stretch my leg. Based on my appearance, however, I should have been placed in the baggage compartment. I was wearing my standard red-dust-hued T-shirt and, because I was wearing a leg brace, matching red-hued shorts. My only luggage was a red-dust-stained, formerly yellow backpack. This was an Aire Afrique flight, where first-class really meant something. Other first-class passengers were dressed to reflect their status. They also—for the most part— qualified for the *Bien engraissé* compliment.

I had never flown first class, of course. I had never experienced a seven-course meal, or had hot, rolled-up, snow-white towels handed to me with silver tongs by a flight attendant who looked like a movie star. (I think we could call them stewardesses back then.) It was a bit embarrassing handing her back a red towel, which I'm sure was simply thrown away. It was also frustrating to be served course after course of fine French cuisine when I had no real appetite. Something was wrong; this should have been a dream come true considering my diet for the past year and the fact that I weighed 135 pounds. I should have been gluttonously gorging myself in a manner that corresponded to my appearance. Instead, I just dozed and tried to make myself inconspicuous.

Arriving at Dulles airport outside of Washington, D.C., in the summer of 1983 prompted some reverse culture shock, even after only having been in Africa for a year. I hobbled outside the terminal to hail a taxi, and was met by the sight of massive automobiles, which were everywhere. I had not seen American vehicles other than the missionaries' Ford truck for a long enough time to be startled by their size. I managed to secure a taxi (another first for me), sat in the front seat (something I later learned that seasoned taxi-hailers do not do), and found my way to the State Plaza hotel, where a room had been reserved for me.

I was back in the States, and to celebrate, I went downstairs to a restaurant in the hotel and promptly did what Americans do: ordered a cheeseburger and fries. Curiously, I once again had little appetite for my meal. This was another dream come true; I should have wolfed down the meal and maybe ordered another one. Even worse, the beer I ordered tasted like water, and I almost sent it back before realizing it was my taste buds that had changed. I had become so accustomed to the full-flavored African beers (the breweries were owned by European brewers), that my American beer seemed tasteless by comparison. After my dinner, I headed back up to my room. It had been a long couple of days, and I had an appointment with the orthopedic surgeon the next morning.

The blood work done on me at the clinic revealed that I had, among other less exciting parasites, malaria. In the US, medical types get all worked up about a simple case of malaria. It was the fifth time for me, so I could not see what all the excitement was about. It turns out that the National Institutes of Health had a keen interest in me, or more specifically, in my blood cells. It had long been suspected that chloroquine, the quinine-based antimalarial drug that we were all taking, was losing its effectiveness in the

CAR. I could have told them that, but they needed proof and here I was, fresh from the CAR with a healthy dose of malaria.

They could not have been happier. I, on the other hand, was laid out on a table with a big hose carrying blood out of one arm, through a centrifuge, and back into my other arm. I recall at one point being certain I was going to die. I had encountered this feeling already in the CAR, the first time I got malaria, when I was all by myself in Bangassou. I had never been sicker in my life. Not only was I convinced that I was going to die, but I really did not care if I did. This time, I knew I was going to die because there was an air bubble, a big one, sliding through the tubing and headed straight for my arm.

Being a Minnesotan in a situation like this creates some internal conflicts. On the one hand, I wanted the nurse to know that I was about to die unless she intervened. On the other hand, I felt self-conscious about drawing attention to myself. Finally, I politely notified her that there was an air bubble about to enter my bloodstream, lodge in my brain, and cause me to die instantly. My friend on my block growing up, Jeff (whose mother was a nurse), had informed me of this fact years earlier. The nurse, however, sauntered over, gave the air bubble a nonchalant flick with her finger, and told me that Jeff had been misinformed. I watched helplessly as the air bubble slid into my arm. But she was right, and I did not die. My blood cells were shipped to the Centers for Disease Control in Atlanta, and I did, in fact, test positive for chloroquine-resistant malaria. This discovery meant that all volunteers and staff stationed in the CAR now had to switch to a sulfa-based antimalarial drug, and that anyone with sulfa allergies had to leave the CAR. All thanks to a pregnant goat.

Following a short stay at George Washington University Hospital, where I received near- celebrity status among the medical students for having *real malaria,* I was finally free to explore our nation's capital, an assignment that I took quite seriously. The Metro in Washington, D.C. was my first real experience using a subway system, and I soon mastered it. Using this ultramodern system, I could go anywhere I wanted in the city. I was popping up all over the place, visiting all the historic sites, museums (including the National Air and Space Museum four times), and restaurants. Where the subway did not go, buses and trains did. I hobbled everywhere and ate my way from Washington to Baltimore. My time spent there would best be described as an eating binge. There were seemingly endless temptations from every type of food imaginable, and I had more per diem than I could possibly spend each day on food. Apparently, per diem rates were based on meals purchased at fancy sit-down restaurants. But I was going for quantity. My restaurant choices were seldom fancier than a Georgetown pizza parlor. Not wanting to keep feeding me, however, the Peace Corps sent me back home to Minnesota, where I was subjected to several weeks of physical therapy. With no more freeloading parasites competing for my meals, I gained nearly forty pounds in three months.

So, when I eventually arrived back in the CAR, in December of 1983, I was rather well- upholstered. As I was being driven back to the Peace Corps transit house, I saw Tom, Pete, and Mac seated outside at the local bar. I had only one thought in mind, jet lag or not, and that was to chuck my gear into the transit house and immediately go have a beer (or several) with my buddies. As I started back down the stairs, however, a gal I had never seen before, one of the new volunteers, was coming up the stairs, and she rudely wanted to introduce herself to me. She smiled and said, "You must be Mark Schultz." Well, who else could I be? Nobody who had been in the country for even a week looked like I did at that moment. First off, I was, as I mentioned, pudgy. I was also attired in brand-new, snug-fitting blue jeans, a brand-new Iowa Hawkeyes jersey (a parting gift from my nieces and nephew), and brand-new sneakers. I looked like it was the first day of school, and there, smiling at me, the only parts of her face not caked with red dust being the two circles behind her glasses, was my future wife. All I saw in her at the time, though, was an obstacle to my rendezvous with my buddies and copious amounts of beer. I muttered something rude and continued my stiff-legged descent to the street. Peg had, herself, just arrived in Bangui from Mobaye on *trafic*. Rather than traveling crammed in the back of the tiny Toyota pickup truck with fifteen other passengers, she had the good fortune of being able to ride in the cab of the truck. Unfortunately, the truck did not have a windshield, which accounted for her raccoon-like appearance.

It was when I returned to my post in Mobaye that the compliments began pouring in. *Bien engraisse´* my admirers would exclaim as they took in my physique. In their eyes, I was touting my wealth and affluence as surely as if I was dripping with gold jewelry. I was showing the world that I had the means to eat as much Western food as I liked, and I also undoubtedly had someone to do my physical work for me. The compliments were short-lived, however. The roundworms, tapeworms, giardia, and amoebas soon moved back into my gut, and once again I had to share my meals with those freeloaders. I have often wondered why The Roundworm Diet has never caught on here in America. I can attest to its effectiveness. It is also inexpensive, and it allows the dieter to keep on eating without gaining weight or performing any dreaded exercise. It sounds like the perfect Hollywood diet to me. Anyone who willingly allows the toxin from *Clostridium botulinum* to be injected into their face so they can look younger should have no problem ingesting a few roundworms in the name of personal vanity. This may be a business opportunity awaiting some enterprising entrepreneur.

IS IT REALLY A PARADOX?

One evening in Bangui, Tom, Pete, Mac, and I were ascending the same stairs where I first encountered Peggy, when we were met by a group of big, hardened, uniformed French soldiers coming down the stairs. When they noticed us, one of them exclaimed, "Look at the Americans! They are all fat!" We got his point. He was articulating, for our benefit, what the French, in general, thought of Americans. We responded by hugging the wall and scampered up the stairs as quickly as our dignity would allow (which was pretty fast). It was hard for us to feel too personally offended by the comment, since we were all seriously underweight at the time, and were having trouble even keeping our trousers up without suspenders (although Tom actually *wore* suspenders). We therefore did not feel too compelled to defend the dignity of our nation.

There is a lot of discussion about the so-called French paradox, which asserts that the French have inexplicably lower rates of obesity and heart disease than Americans do, even though the French diet tends to be much higher in fat. While I have done no serious research of my own on the subject, I have made some *observations*. (Observations are much less time-consuming than research, and one is not burdened by the need to be accurate or correct.) At the heart of the matter is, I believe, the preference by the French for fresh, whole foods. The French paradox can only be a paradox if what the French are doing contradicts a known fact—that eating fat causes people to become fat. This *conventional wisdom*, handed down from on high for the past forty years, is being questioned by folks who are much smarter than I am; and I tend to agree with them.

My Swedish grandparents ate a very similar high-fat, French-type diet their entire lives. Factory-made foods simply had no place in Grandma's farm kitchen. Sure, she would buy me the eight-packs of single-serving sugared cereals; but that was because I was special. My two favorites were Sugar Pops and Sugar Smacks. This was back before the marketers wisely changed the respective names to Corn Pops and Honey Smacks. Rather than remove the sugar from their products, they simply removed it from their names. Otherwise, if there was cereal on my grandparents' table it would have been Corn Flakes, served with cream. What I recall most about breakfast at the farm, however, was a spread of cured meats, fish, and cheeses, some of Grandma's homemade bread, and donuts that had been fried in lard. There were whole anchovies, head-down, lining a glass jar. There was pickled herring, and Grandpa loved to boil up some of the smallest sunfish that we kept just for breakfast. This was what we ate after we had come in from an hour or two of farm chores. Virtually everyone from that era ate a diet that was based on whole foods and plenty of fat. The culprit that is re-emerging, the one that our mothers said would make us fat but had no idea why: *sugar*.

I ate quite a bit of French cuisine in Africa (and in France). I, in fact, became rather well-known for my uncanny ability to show up just before the noon meal at the residences that had the best cooks. I found that the time and care that the French took to prepare fresh food was worthwhile and satisfying. They even made cow brains delicious, for Pete's sake! Seldom seen at their tables were bags of chips, store-bought cookies, or any of the other processed foods that line the shelves in the middle sections of our supermarkets. That is not to say that the French avoided sweets. They had the good sense to serve chocolate for breakfast, for example. Sweets were a treat, though, and not a way of life. The French folks that I hung out with ate real, whole, very well-prepared food—and plenty of it. What they also did differently was savor their meals and not eat like we tend to do, which is more like an eating contest. Julia Child once said: "In France, cooking is a serious art form and a national sport". There is also the issue of physical activity, such as walking or biking to the local market rather than driving there. A village lifestyle perhaps makes obtaining fresh, local foods, and getting exercise in the fresh air much easier, as well as having less stress and more *joie de vivre*. But it is certainly also obtainable in urban areas.

If there is a French paradox, I think it is less about their high-fat diet, and more about their tobacco use. Most of the French people I met used tobacco products. It may be, perhaps, that a wholesome diet goes a long way toward warding off even the ill effects of smoking. French cuisine is firmly entrenched in their culture, and this helps them resist changes to it. I saw very few American franchise restaurants when I was in France in 1984. It has likely changed since then, but I suspect that peddling American food is still a tough sell in France.

NEVER HAS IT BEEN HARDER TO BE CONTENT

Tristan Jones, the Welsh sailor and adventurer, was one of my favorite writers. This quote is a bit long, but I want to share with you the observations he made in the 1960s while he was visiting the island of Formentera off the eastern coast of Spain. This is an excerpt from his book, *Seagulls in my Soup*.

> The Formenterans appeared to be among the healthiest folk I have ever seen, and it's a fact that at the far southern end of the island there was a small hamlet, near Cape Berberia, where there were, out of a population of around 200, thirty-odd persons over the age of 100 years. It was not a rare thing to see one of the ancient men, small and sunburned, dressed all in black, scrambling up the 500-foot high cliffs of the cape as sure-footed and agile as a goat-with a full-sized turtle, weighing 100 pounds or more, slung over his shoulder. I have seen several places like this where people live long and die happy. I have often thought about the reason for this. Is it diet? Is it something in the water? Is it something inherited? After having observed these folks in places as far apart as Turkey and Bolivia, I conclude that there are a few traits these ancients have in common: They live without haste. They have just enough for their own needs, and they want no more. They are usually jealous of what they have, but they do not covet. Neither do

> they resent growing old. In the main they accept it
> as part of life, but not with sorrow, because another
> thing the long-lived folk have in common the world
> over is a strong faith in the hereafter…

I wanted to share Tristan's thoughts because I had observed much the same thing while living in the CAR. My first post, Bangassou, was a good 150 kilometers upstream from Mobaye, on a branch of the Oubangui River, called the Mbomou. Like Mobaye, Bangassou was a remnant of the bygone days of French colonialism, when goods traveled much more effectively by water than over land. The major towns, therefore, were generally built along the major rivers. Unlike the terrain around Mobaye, Bangassou was situated in a region of spectacular rainforest. I was sent to Bangassou because there had been a fisheries volunteer there before me, and I was to be her replacement. There was a fundamental problem with this posting, however, which became immediately apparent; in a rainforest, I could not build the types of ponds we had been taught to build.

For the past twenty years, the aquaculture program in the CAR had been administered by the United Nations Food and Agricultural Organization (FAO). Their program was based on groundwater ponds, which were simply some holes dug in wet areas, and groundwater seeped in to fill them. The main problem with this type of pond is that it doesn't work.

Under the tutelage of the FAO, Central African extension agents were selected to represent each area served by the program. There was a main hatchery and fisheries station located in Bambari, about 200 kilometers northwest of Mobaye, and 300 kilometers from Bangassou, where once or twice a year the FAO sponsored a training session for the agents. The fisheries program, as administered by the FAO, was an all-too-stereotypical government aid program. Paid European project managers lived in the houses at the fisheries station, some of the finest houses east of Bangui.

These managers, generally French or Belgian, were European versions of Peace Corps volunteers—except for being better funded. Compared to us, they lived in luxury. Under their management, Central African agents were selected from villages within the service area of the station, with the only prerequisite being that they could read at a third-grade level. During a training session, the agents would be given a new manual on how to dig a hole in the ground and how to stock the hole with fingerlings obtained from the fisheries station. The station was the heart of the operation. Without it, there would be no FAO fisheries program, because farmers were incapable of stocking their own ponds with their own fingerlings, and because the ponds could not be drained or properly managed.

The FAO program was doomed to fail. Despite the FAO's twenty-year presence, the farmers were not having success raising a decent amount of fish in their ponds. The instruction manuals handed out during the training sessions showed the agents how to dig a hole in the ground anywhere there was groundwater just below the surface, which was inevitably alongside a small stream in the forest. Using a short, hand-forged shovel or hoe to dig a pond in the mud and roots was back-breaking work, and the ponds were, by necessity, quite small. The holes filled with water as they were being dug, making them also quite shallow. When there were enough holes to put fish in, the agents scheduled a shipment of tilapia fingerlings from the station in Bambari. When the truck arrived with aerated tanks filled with fingerlings, he would fill five-gallon plastic jerry cans with water and fingerlings, sling two of them over the rack on the back of his bicycle in a burlap sack, and pedal off to the remote pond sites.

The prime motivator for this hard work was not the promise of a bountiful harvest. For the agents, it was the gift of a bicycle, the small stipend that he received, and the prestige of his position. For the typical villager, there was little hope of ever obtaining a mode of transportation more refined than a bicycle. Even a bicycle was out of reach for most villagers, so to have one given to him by the FAO was a huge motivator for an agent. For the farmers, the rewards were few, other than the possibility of the FAO donating a shovel or two or a wheelbarrow for the village to share. I believe that many of them undertook the effort of digging and harvesting these ponds simply because there was still a deep-seated *patron* system in the CAR, where white patrons made the rules and they were obeyed, whether they made sense or not.

When the agent announced the date for the arrival of the fingerling truck, it was time for the farmers to harvest their ponds. The women of the village were assigned the task of draining the ponds, which consisted of using their wash basins as scoops to toss out the water. I participated in one of these drainages once, to see for myself how much work was involved in draining a pond. After about five minutes of scooping and tossing out water, I felt as though I had just run five miles in chest waders. It was backbreaking labor. We stood knee-deep in muck in the tropical heat and humidity trying futilely to gain headway on the water that was seeping back into the pond almost as quickly as it was being scooped out. While the women tossed out the water, the men would wade around in the fluid muck, frantically picking up any fish they could find and putting them in baskets. The harvest was always heartbreakingly meager and often exceeded by the frog harvest.

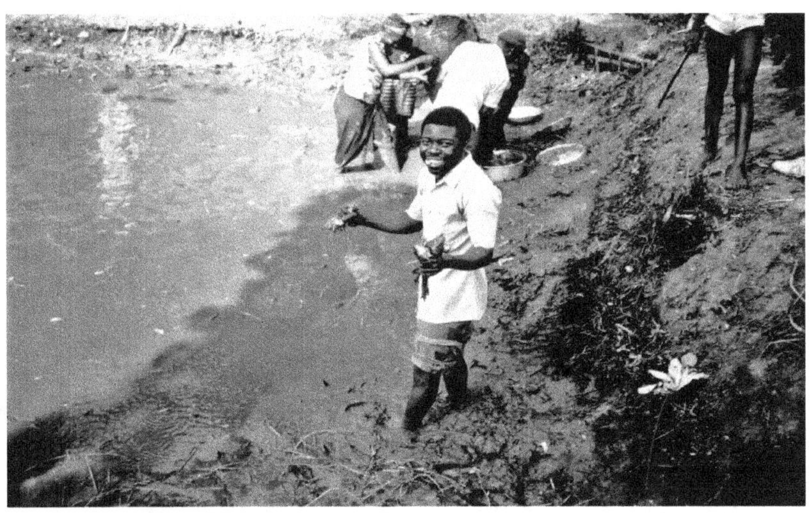

Bangassou pond drainage and a farmer happy with his frog harvest

Besides being small and terribly labor-intensive, the main fault of groundwater ponds was that they could never be fully drained, and therefore never fully harvested. Wild predatory fish could not be eradicated and would eat most of the highly vulnerable stocked fingerlings. A typical harvest yielded a paltry two pounds of stunted fish to show for six months of growth. After twenty years, this was the state of aquaculture in the CAR. But that was all about to change.

Unlike my predecessor, who had bought into this established FAO model, our group was the inaugural product of a whole new approach to aquaculture developed by the University of Oklahoma's Peace Corps Fisheries Training Program. The program is probably best described as ten intensive weeks of a combination of boot camp, Outward Bound, and brainwashing, with one goal: to make us all disciples of the diversion pond, self-reliance, and the profit motive. Our mission was to work only with ponds that could be fully drained, and therefore to concentrate our efforts only on the sites that had the best potential for proper pond construction. This program was designed to turn the FAO model on its ear. We either bought into it and worked hard to prove that we were up to the task of implementing it or we were on the next flight home without even a goodbye to our fellow trainees.

I was miserable in Bangassou, and not just because I was lonelier and more homesick than I had ever been in my life and had my first case of malaria, which convinced me that I was going to die. I was miserable because there was not a single pond site anywhere in my region suitable for the type of pond culture we were taught to promote. Tom was miserable in Alindao for other reasons. Being closer to Bambari, and the FAO fiefdom, he was being controlled by a big, intimidating, unpleasant Central African petty bureaucrat named Leonard. He was funded by the FAO to run the district that Tom had been assigned to, and he saw Tom as a threat to his authority. FAO still operated like they were going to be running the fisheries program for the next twenty years; but their days were numbered. The US Agency for International Development (USAID) would soon be taking over the funding of the fisheries program, and it was *our* approach to aquaculture that they embraced.

Tom and I began commiserating by letter, which we could do with a fair amount of regularity due to the flow of traffic—mostly by the Catholic missions—between Alindao and Bangassou, and the fact that we both had a lot of time on our hands. We hatched a scheme that he and I should divide Tom's district, the Basse-Kotto, in half. He would work the fifty-kilometer radius around Alindao in the north, and I would work the southern half. We only had to convince our director that this was a good idea. We found, initially, that directors generally are not too fond of being informed by new, cocky volunteers that they had made a posting error. Paul, our director, did not necessarily share our zeal for diversion ponds. To his credit, though, Paul agreed to come out to the Basse-Kotto and he, Tom, and I made a grand tour, from Alindao to Mobaye. It was mostly the spectacular terrain that finally sold him on the idea. The Basse-Kotto was a pond builder's paradise, with nearly every village having a gently sloping valley nearby, with grassy slopes and a reliably flowing stream at the bottom. Besides the obvious benefits of the terrain, I think Paul admired the passion and enthusiasm that Tom and I displayed, which was partly due to our indoctrination, partly because we both needed each other, and partly because we, too, were blown away by the majesty of the Basse-Kotto.

That was how I got to Mobaye. Now we will go back to Bangassou, because that is where the event that made me think about Tristan Jones' observations took place. My agent at the time had informed me that the Chef de Village of a remote village out east had requested a site visit from us to assess the feasibility of raising tilapia in his village. So, early one dry season morning the two of us took off on my motorcycle on the Trans-African Highway going east toward Sudan. By *highway*, I mean a deeply rutted, single-lane dirt road that became impassable for much of the rainy season due to the need to ford small rivers that became big rivers, and ruts that became canyon-like. By *motorcycle*, I mean a 125 cc Suzuki dirt bike, the kind that dads here in northern Minnesota buy for their kids to ride, before they learn to ride a real motorcycle. Two adults could fit on it but being of the opposite sex would have been advantageous; especially as we climbed in and out of three-foot deep ravines.

We traveled east for what seemed like a very long time until my agent motioned for me to turn north on a narrow path. We slowly made our way along this forest trail, and then my agent told me to stop. From there we had to travel on foot. I had the sense that we were walking into another world, back in time, as the hard-packed footpath wove around the deeply buttressed bases of massive tropical hardwoods, in a forest that had likely been a forest for eons. I felt like I was in a place as remote as any left on earth. We had just spent a couple of hours traveling on a modern, powerful machine to get to this narrow path where no machine could go or had ever gone.

Anyone who lived in the village we were about to visit would need to walk at least a day and a half just to get to Bangassou, and the Chef de Village we were going to visit had done just that when he came to request a visit from us. It was actually me he had come to see. He had heard that there was a new patron in town to administer the aquaculture program, so he came to meet me and personally ask if I would visit his village. I will never forget the morning this wiry old man, dressed in tattered clothes and plastic shoes, knocked politely on my door, with his hat in his hands—mainly because of the shameful way I treated him. I had grown accustomed to being asked for money or gifts by some of the townspeople. One of the most popular sayings in Sango is *mu na mbi*, which means *give it to me*. I was already becoming cynical, and I callously assumed that he was there to ask for money. What a rude dope I was, and although I have done lots of shameful things in my life, turning that fine man away from my door ranks way up there as one I still think of nearly 4 decades later.

Now, having traveled the same road that he had traveled to visit the Great Patron, I imagined his confusion and disappointment at my behavior. The wisdom of the saying, "Walk a mile in my shoes," hit home. When we finally broke into a clearing in the deep, ancient forest village that was their home, I was made to feel like my visit was the highest honor they could possibly have been awarded, even if I was just an ungrateful kid from Minnesota who had much to learn about human decency. I was about to get a huge dose of it.

The chef came to greet us carrying his most prized possession, a battery-operated shortwave radio. After thanking me for my visit, he proudly showed us around the village and, as expected, a very inappropriate site to construct a pond. I had to explain to him, mostly through my agent as interpreter, that it would be unfeasible not only to build a pond, but also to supply fingerlings to such a remote location. Rather than being upset or disappointed, the villagers accepted the verdict of the wise Patron and we spent the remainder of the visit sitting under a tree eating fresh fruit.

What struck me then and has stuck with me ever since then, was the feeling that I had just met some of the most Christian people in my life; and yet I knew that no mission had influenced these people of the forest. They had likely never been inside of a church, and yet they were some of the kindest, most generous and caring people on Earth. I then realized that *Christian* was perhaps not the proper label. These were people of God who knew right from wrong as easily as they knew how to breathe; and since any breath they took could be their last, they lived with that awareness and gratefulness. They packed all the living they possibly could into the lives that they were given. In this remote forest clearing there would be no medical treatment for any ailment. A ruptured appendix, an accident with a machete, a complication during childbirth, or any of the issues that would be routine for us would mean certain death for them. Central Africans routinely witnessed suffering and death from diseases, but they did not despair, blame, complain, covet, or partake in the major sins that seem to afflict those of us back in *civilization*. They were content.

I was to experience the feeling many times in the CAR that it was people like me, those of us with so many possessions, who were missing out on the true joy of living. We have medical advances on our side to keep us alive for far more years than most villagers. But from what I saw, they knew how to pack more life into a day than we ever could. The villagers had only each other, and so they found joy in each other. I saw and heard more laughter from the villagers than I would have imagined possible, since it seemed to me that they should have little to laugh about, given their poverty and daily reminders of their own mortality. To think back on an ancient villager humbly greeting me and have them feel so honored to have me take their calloused, gnarled hand, gives me the incentive to work harder at being a better person—one who may come closer to being worthy of their handshake.

I recall my upbringing in the Lutheran church and, prior to taking communion, hearing the pastor's words, "We are by nature sinful and unclean." The Lutheran church, at least at that time, was not big on building self-esteem. What Tristan Jones and I had observed in some of the poorest corners of the world contradicts this edict. I believe the *sinful and unclean* part is man- made, and not part of our nature. It is our lust for possessions, for the money to buy those possessions, and the lust for power that comes from having all that money, that gets the *sinful and unclean* part to kick in.

In one of my favorite movies, *The Gods Must be Crazy*, the pilot of a small plane tosses an empty Coca-Cola bottle out of his window over a remote region in southern Africa, where it happens to land near a village of *San*, or Bushmen. Prior to the arrival of the bottle, the villagers are shown to be living contented lives. The bottle, however, soon becomes a coveted object and envy, jealousy, greed, and finally violence threatens to destroy their way of life. The hero of the story sees that the only way the village can return to its former peaceful, contented existence, is for the bottle to be destroyed by throwing it off the edge of the world (the ocean). What he encounters on this journey is hilarious and filled with just the type of slapstick comedy that Central Africans would love.

Several years ago, I was relaxing in the sauna on a cold winter day, studying a seed catalog, when Peg stepped in to join me. She said she had been delayed in the house by an interesting discussion on public radio about what it means to be happy. She then asked me how I would describe happiness. I thought for a bit, and said, "To me, it means being content." The isolated villagers in the CAR were content. Thinking back, my friends and I on our block growing up in single-income families with modest homes, with little more than each other, a glove and a bat across our handlebars, and our imaginations, were content. Young children, even today, before they learn to covet the endless array of stuff that they are bombarded with, are content. It was during the Time of Great Change, when corporations mastered their marketing skills, that being content became so difficult to maintain past the third grade.

One Sunday morning, Peg had written a quote from our pastor on a corner of the church bulletin during one of his sermons, and she stuck it on our refrigerator. More than ten years later, it is still up there. It says: "Never has it been harder to be content." Making a purchase makes us happy. Purchasing things that make our children happy makes us happy. But the happiness that a purchase stimulates is short-lived. Soon there is a new, better model of what we bought, and then we want that too (which version of the iPhone are we on now?). It seems to me that, with every purchase we make, every time we covet some new object, we move ourselves one notch further from the point in our lives where we were content to have our basic needs met, to simply enjoy the company of others, and to be loved.

It is not surprising that our nation is experiencing an epidemic of drug addiction. The opposite of addiction, as I see it, is not sobriety; it is *connection* with each other and with the natural world that sustains us.

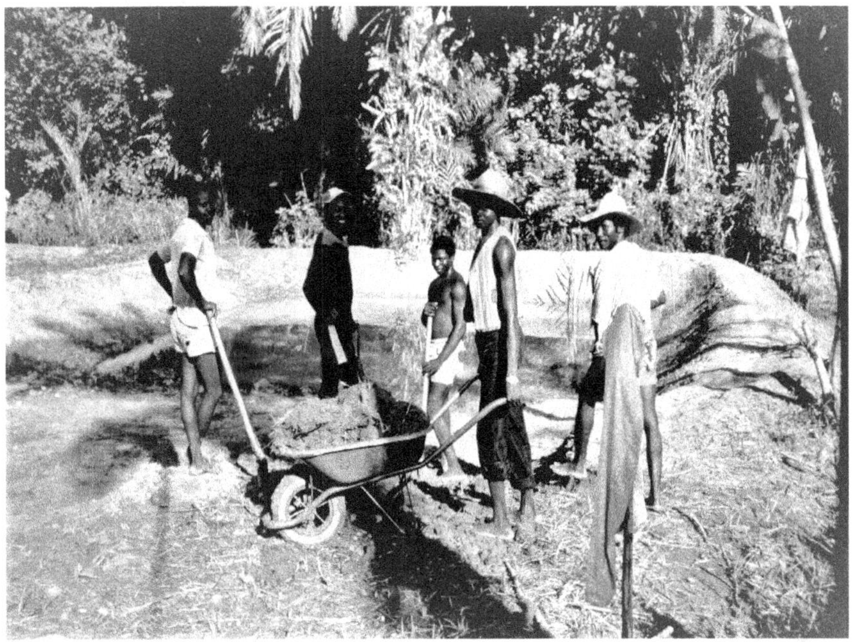

Villagers working together to accomplish great things- and enjoy doing it

IT JUST SEEMS TO RUN BETTER

My moto was my life. Sure, I commandeered the program's Toyota truck more than my share of the time; but for the daily travels to the villages, I depended on my moto. Although it was a kid's bike by American standards, Central Africans would marvel at this sleek machine as I cruised by, and I would hear them exclaim, "Suzuki Cross! Cent-Vingt-Cinq!" The neighbor kids loved to come over and sit on it, much as an American kid might get a kick out of climbing into the cockpit of a fighter jet.

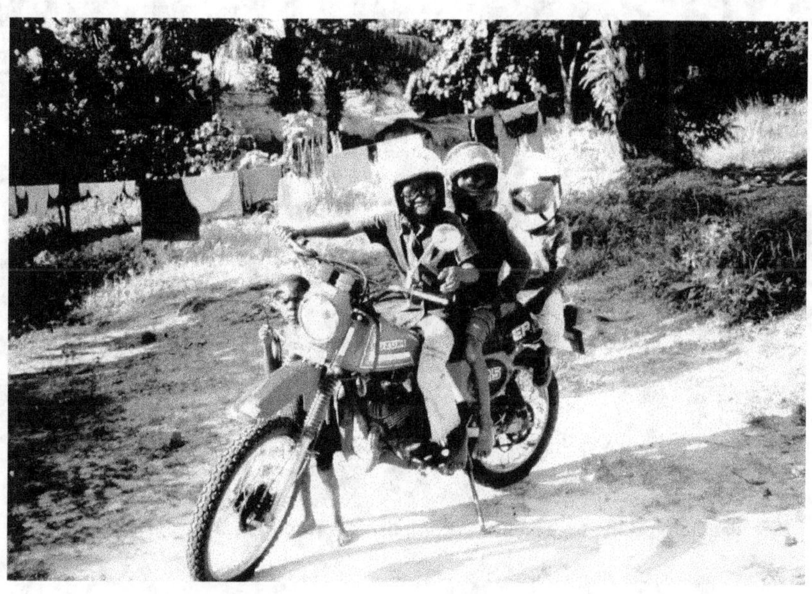

The neighbor kids on my moto- wearing helmets of course

So, every Sunday afternoon—since Sunday was technically my only day off—I performed the same ritual on my moto. I would wheel it out to the front steps of my house, heat some water, get out a bar of soap, some kerosene, an old toothbrush, oil, rags, and wrenches, and perform my Sunday maintenance. During the week, this little workhorse had gotten me through streambeds and ravines, bounced along rock-strewn paths, passed through clouds of dust, and de-feathered the odd chicken. So, I got to work washing the red dust from the surfaces and cleaning grime from the hard-to-reach places using the toothbrush dipped in kerosene. I oiled all the moving parts: the chain, cables, linkages, and sprockets. I tightened all the nuts that had vibrated loose during the previous week. I pulled and cleaned the spark plug, and occasionally pulled the cylinder head and scraped off the accumulated carbon deposits.

When the session was complete, I would hop on the sparkling machine and take it for a spin down to Centre Ville and back. What always struck me was that, even though this was the same moto and I had not replaced any of the parts, it felt like I was riding a new machine. It just seemed to run better.

When a new batch of fisheries trainees arrived to replace our group, I was asked to teach the motorcycle and truck maintenance course at the training facility in M'Baiki. As a bit of cruel irony, while on my journey from Bangui to M'Baiki, the little view window at the bottom of the two-cycle oil reservoir that allows the operator to see the oil level vibrated loose, allowing the two- cycle oil to drain out. Now that I think about it, there were two ironic events occurring here. It was ironic to find the teacher of the maintenance course broken down along the roadside. It was also ironic that the little view window that existed to prevent what had happened actually caused the problem. The engine made a sickening, screeching sound as the piston rings fused to the cylinder wall, and I coasted to the edge of the road. I did not have to ponder my predicament long. A Peace Corps truck, filled with my future students, pulled over to meet their instructor. As we loaded my moto into the back of the truck, I explained that, on the bright side, they were going to have the opportunity to learn how to rebuild an engine.

During our training sessions, to reinforce the importance of maintenance, I told my students about the feeling I experienced during my test rides. I said to them, "I can't quite put my finger on it, but it just seems to run better."

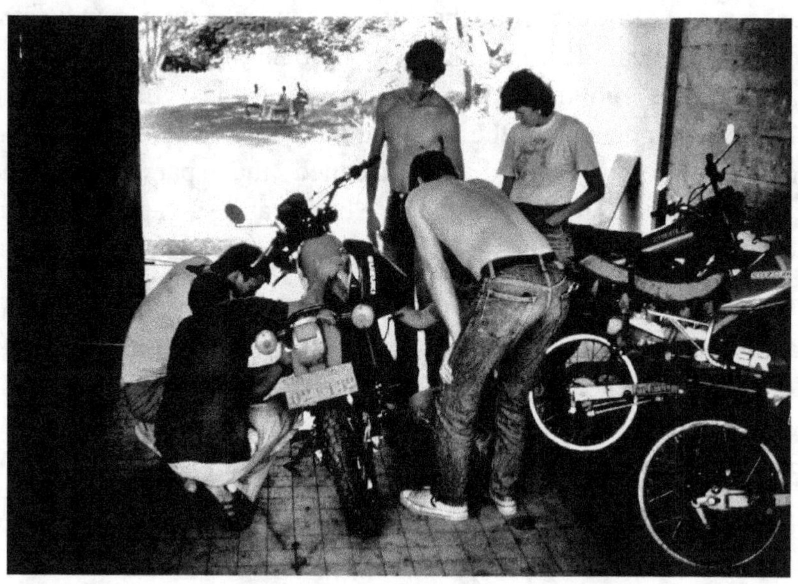

Moto maintenance in M'Baiki-1984

After being at his post for a few months, I ran into one of the new volunteers in Bangui. He excitedly came up to me and exclaimed: "You were right. I felt it. It just seemed to run better!" I told this story once to Peg's Sunday school class when I was filling in for her, because of the similar feeling I get after a Sunday church service. During the week, we are out there being jostled along the rock-strewn, muddy, deeply rutted road of life. If this goes on, week after week, without pausing to get cleaned, tightened, and lubricated, we eventually start running around with a few screws loose. Attending a weekly service usually does it for me. Whatever it is for others, it must be something. For Central African villagers, it was having each other, and the evenings spent visiting around the fire. It might be time spent alone in a wilderness, paddling a canoe, or being propelled across the water under the power of the wind. For some, it could be something as simple as tending a garden.

THE WELLNESS CENTER

I knew of folks living in Mobaye who grew produce in raised bed gardens. I dined on their produce nearly every day, but I was too single-minded in those days to be curious about those gardens. Back then, it was all about building and maintaining fishponds. Looking back, I regret not learning more about those gardeners. Come to think of it, I also regret not being curious about how Central African women in Mobaye could create crispy, tender baguettes in simple, outdoor, mud-brick ovens. The produce on display at the morning market would be the envy of any American farmers market. There were peppers, tomatoes, onions, garlic, celery (the leafy variety), carrots, melons, and a vast array of greens of some sort generally available year-round. I figured these gardening techniques were introduced by the French and sustained by the Catholic mission. I now wonder about how they created their rich, compost-based soil. Those gardeners were organic well before being organic was cool.

I know now just what I would do if I had the opportunity to go back to Mobaye as a gardening volunteer. First, I would bring along our product, the Garden Stream™ (which we will discuss in detail later), to automate the watering of self-watering planters. I would install rain barrels for the primary water supply, and I would promote composting. I would also construct raised beds from corrugated metal and use chopped leaves to build living soil. Then I would concentrate on growing, besides all the regular produce, melons. Watermelon and other melons were in high demand, especially by the Lebanese merchants and other expatriates. Central Africans were also fond of them, but melons were rather expensive to grow and difficult to water adequately. Using our container system, they would use about twenty percent of the water of conventional gardening, and there are now compact plant varieties which are better suited to container gardening. That would have been fun back then. Unfortunately, it would not be fun, or safe, to work over there now.

Now that we are passionate gardeners, I understand how important gardening is to our physical and spiritual health. Dining on absolutely-fresh, nutrient-dense produce is obviously good for our bodies. But tending a garden also grounds and centers us. To nurture a garden is to watch a miracle unfold in slow motion. A garden reminds us of our ties to the natural world that sustains us. Whenever I find myself disturbed or perplexed by something, I am drawn to our garden. Next thing I know, I am wandering around the raised beds, stopping to pull an uninvited weed, doing some thinning, or simply looking to see if I can detect any growth since my last visit, perhaps three hours earlier. I may be oversimplifying a complex cultural problem, but I believe that something as simple as tending a garden could give purpose and meaning to life for someone who is feeling lost. We all need a reason to want to get up and out of bed in the morning. For some, it could be to get out and check on their miracle.

ACROSS THE RIVER

Mobutu Sese Seko, the self-proclaimed Emperor-for-Life of what was then Zaire, grew up in a small village called Gbadolite, about twenty-five kilometers southwest of Mobaye. In the early 1980s, Mobutu was at the height of his wealth and power. To show it off, he turned his ancestral home into a fantasyland, including a palace, cathedral (with a moat and Chinese swans), a hospital, hotels, a supermarket, and several international aid projects. Since it was so close to Mobaye, it was an irresistible temptation to sneak across the border and visit Gbadolite. It was a bit like taking guests to Disney World when they visited us while we lived in Florida. In fact, it was a lot like Disney World (or, perhaps more accurately, *The Twilight Zone*). So, whenever we were visited by volunteers from other regions, we were expected to take them to Gbadolite.

There were a few issues with such a trip, since we had to transport our motos across the Oubangui in dug-out canoes, and we were technically entering a foreign country without authorization or passports. Having to explain how my moto ended up on the bottom of the river to my director was one concern, the other was of him having to disrupt his day to negotiate a prisoner exchange. It was illegal, of course, for us to enter a foreign nation without passports or permission, but there was ice cream and real butter, mayonnaise, and Green Giant Niblets corn just over there, across the river, twenty-five kilometers away, in an air-conditioned supermarket! It was well worth the risk. So, with a few extra bills tucked away to appease any meddling soldiers, we lifted our motos into the most stable dug-out canoes we could find, and away we went to Gbadolite.

This monument to the excesses of a dictator who had become one of the world's wealthiest men partly due to the generosity of donor nations (like ours) included one of the most unlikely aid projects imaginable: a dairy. Out of curiosity, we went to visit this operation on one of our clandestine trips to Gbadolite. I do not recall which nation, or nations, got snookered into funding such an inappropriate project in Equatorial Africa, but I do recall meeting some fellow Minnesotans who were there legally. Apparently, they were visiting a mission in Zaire, and the dairy and associated beef cattle operation was part of their tour. It was certainly a surprise to run into fellow Minnesotans in such a remote and strange location. The presence of this dairy proved to me that anything is possible if one has unlimited funds. If the Emperor-for-Life wants a dairy, he gets one.

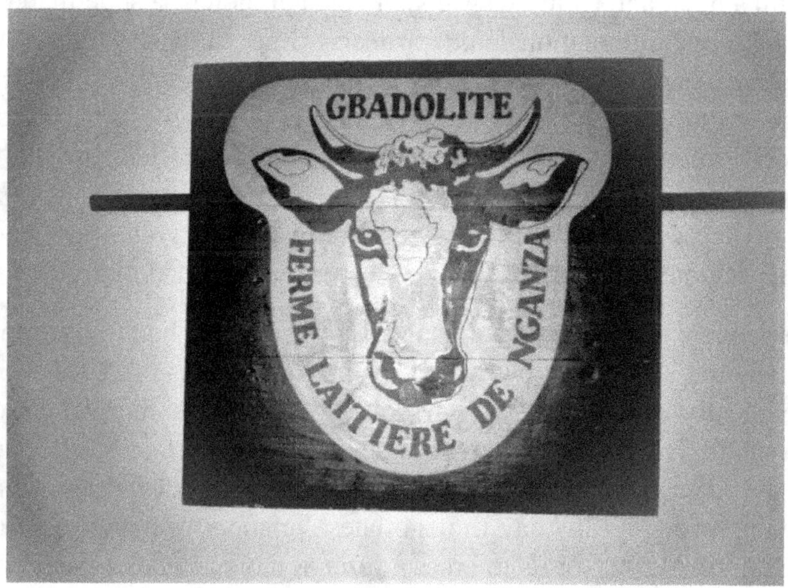

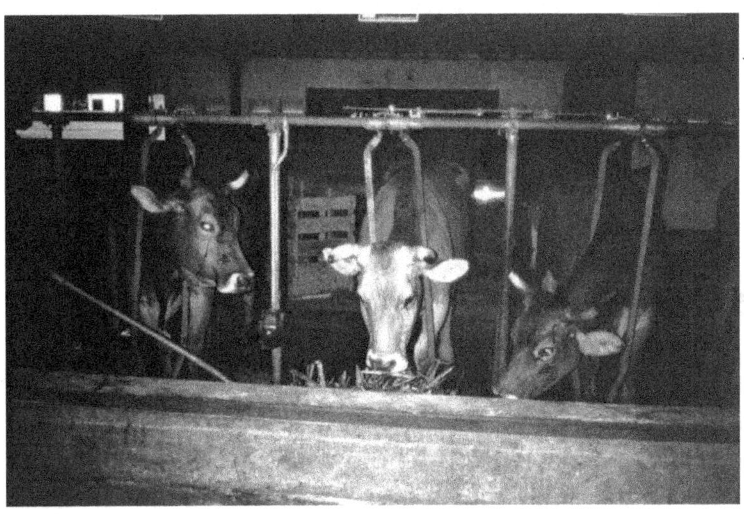

A dairy in the heart of Africa?

The closest Central Africans got to consuming dairy products was when they added canned sweetened condensed milk to their coffee, something the beignet ladies offered to their customers. Otherwise, dairy products were considered a Western food that was out of reach for the average villager and had never been a part of their culture. It was rumored that among the nomadic cattle herders, the Mbororo, yogurt was consumed as part of their diet. I imagine a brave herder would occasionally dare to sneak a few squirts of milk from a long-horned cow into a gourd, and it would become yogurt by the end of the day. This would only have been consumed among themselves and was not something to be sold in the markets. I suspect there was a degree of lactose intolerance by the Central Africans. Despite the absence of dairy products, however, there was no indication of osteoporosis. In fact, these folks had some of the strongest, straightest backs I have ever seen. They could easily support fifty pounds of goods on their heads while using their arms mostly just to balance the load, and the elderly were just as capable as the young. Central Africans also had some of the whitest, straightest teeth imaginable. They were certainly getting adequate calcium from somewhere, but it was most likely from the nutritious greens and not from milk.

APPROPRIATE TECHNOLOGY

Peg and I entered the small-business world by selling equipment to make home food processing more efficient. We sold things like food grinders, vegetable strainers, sausage stuffers, and dehydrators. These were simple machines, for the most part hand-operated, that made an unpleasant task more pleasant and efficient. In America, with anything we want (even our food) now available to us from the comfort of our own homes, any time-consuming, labor-intensive task will soon be abandoned in favor of a more pleasant alternative. Take gardening for example. If what we can grow can be purchased, and if we are not enjoying the time and work involved in gardening, most of us will quit doing it. Our job is to remove the *dread factor*, to make it fun, easy, and rewarding, and to develop a degree of self-reliance.

The Central Africans could not just quit growing their own food because it was not fun anymore. What they did was take an appropriate technology approach to living. Africans, by necessity, are experts at appropriate technology. They use what is available to them to make the tasks that sustain them as efficient as possible, and without spending money that they do not have anyway. As an example, I recall my first exposure to raised-bed gardening. Tom and I were in northern Gabon, making our way to Cameroon, and stopped to dine at a local bar and restaurant that had been recommended to us by our friends. The owner, a local man, grew most of his own produce in about a dozen raised beds.

What was striking about his raised beds was his choice of material for his borders, which consisted of hundreds of inverted beer and wine bottles with their necks buried in the ground. He did not have a building supply store nearby, or likely the money to purchase expensive planks or metal to use as borders. Besides, being on the equator, most wood in contact with the ground would become termite food in no time. However, he had lots and lots of beer bottles. I thought it was brilliant, and I was even more amazed when the skies opened-up, in typical rainy season fashion, and there was a torrential downpour. The ground surrounding the raised beds was soon flooded, but the beds themselves remained high and dry—or at least not flooded. The owner explained that this was called the *French Intensive Method* of gardening, and it was the best way to raise produce in the tropics. One reason for this had just been demonstrated to us. The others, he explained, were that he could fill the beds with rich compost, and therefore grow plants much more densely than he could in the nutrient-poor, brick-hard laterite soil. There was also less pest control, less weeding, less watering, and less tilling. This was African-style appropriate technology.

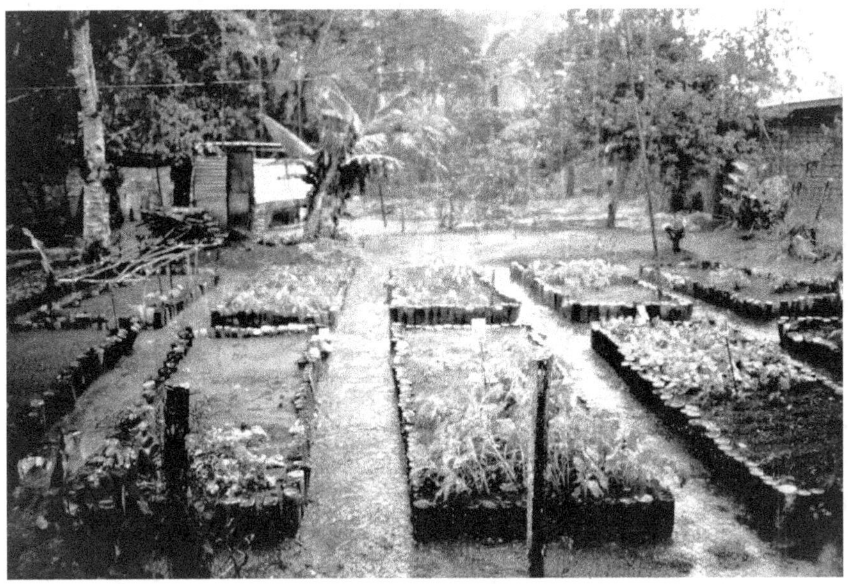

Beer bottle bordered raised beds during a downpour

As another example, I was returning to Mobaye from Alindao once on trafic, which was something I did my best to avoid. All I can think of is that I had gotten a lift to Alindao from the Lebanese merchants to visit Tom, but for some reason I was not able to ride back to Mobaye with them. Trafic was something other volunteers took, but not us. But here I was, packed with the other fifteen or so passengers on my four inches of wooden bench space in the back of a tiny Toyota pickup truck.

The owners of such trucks made a decent living by operating these transport services. When the benches were full, the driver would slam on the brakes to compact his load and make room for another half dozen passengers. This particular driver had a fondness for palm wine that I found disturbing. At every passenger stop, there was the inevitable palm wine vendor operating from the shade of a mango tree. As his associate assisted passengers, the driver would down another quick gourd-full of palm wine. After a few stops I noticed a trend: His speed increased in direct proportion to his consumption of palm wine.

About halfway to Mobaye, while rocketing along the rutted road, we got a flat tire, which was a common occurrence, and we careened to a stop. While the driver consumed yet another gourdful of palm wine, his associate removed the tire and inner tube, and disappeared into the forest. He came back with some latex that he had tapped from a tree, applied a patch using it, pumped up the tire, remounted it, and away we went. I do not know whether this is possible or not. All I know is that I saw it happen. By now, I feared for my life, so I asked to be dropped off at the next village and made no attempt to get a partial refund on my fare to Mobaye. I had to wait a few hours before I could flag down a transport truck headed to Mobaye and ride the rest of the way perched on top of rattling crates of beer and Coca-Cola, some of which, no doubt, were destined for Henri's boutique.

Tom and I, while traveling together in the project truck, were once the first responders, just outside of Alindao, to an awful scene where one of these overloaded trucks had overturned due to excessive speed that most likely involved palm wine. We transported some of the most critically injured passengers to the mission in Alindao, where one woman with a severely broken wrist died, most likely from the loss of blood.

The finest example of appropriate technology I saw was the village house; at least, it was once again becoming a fine example while I was there. A brief history of the CAR is required here, not because I am anywhere near an expert on the subject, but because it has to do with house construction and with the absurdity of some governments and their leaders.

Back in the early- to mid-twentieth century, one of the commodities that the French were extracting from the CAR was cotton. The labor force consisted, of course, of Central African villagers, who were informed by their patrons that the cotton quotas needed to be increased. Stepping up the production of cotton, under the oppressive heat and humidity of Equatorial Africa, was undoubtedly a hellish experience. I knew what it was like to work for just five hours in the heat, and I had Henri's ice-cold Coca-Cola and Celestin's hot meals to look forward to. These folks were likely treated little better than slaves.

Born from this oppression, champion for independence Barthélemy Boganda became the first prime minister of the newly formed Central African Republic in 1959. He died shortly thereafter, in a plane crash that was still, in the 1980s, talked about by Central Africans as if it had occurred the week before. Anyone who has visited the CAR cannot help but wonder what may have been had that plane not crashed. Perhaps it would be a nation where village women do not necessarily die from a broken wrist.

David Dacko, Boganda's cousin, then became the first president of the CAR, and he governed until the last day of 1965, when Jean-Bédal Bokassa overthrew him as part of a New Year's Eve celebration that must have gotten out of hand. The only reason the world knows so little about Bokassa is because another character, Idi Amin, was doing even more outrageous things at the same time in Uganda. To assure job security, Bokassa declared himself President-for-Life in 1972. When that wasn't enough, he renamed the country the Central African Empire, and declared himself *Emperor*-for-Life, complete with an elaborate coronation and his own Arc de Triomphe to march through. Even France, the puppet-string holder, was becoming embarrassed. When one hundred students were murdered for protesting the requirement that all students must buy and wear expensive uniforms made in a factory owned by one of Bokassa's wives, the puppet strings had to be cut. He was tried for murder (but acquitted on cannibalism charges) and sentenced to solitary confinement. In 1993 he was freed and lived-out his final days in Bangui.

The reason I bring up Bokassa here is because one of his many absurd decrees was to ban the construction of the traditional round home. Because he had been to France, where he had seen rectangular houses, Bokassa saw round ones as a sign of backwardness. To look modern, all houses now had to be rectangular. It did not matter that the round hut was, for the Central African environment, perfection in design, or that there was no one in the CAR who had ever built a rectangular house. From now on, all villages were to resemble suburban Paris. But the round, mud-walled hut was a thing of beauty both in its appearance and in its practicality.

The round hut was appropriate technology at its finest. Perhaps one of its best features, according to the villagers, was the fact that there were no corners and therefore no places for evil spirits to hide. Rectangles, gable ends, ridge beams, and rafter ties were all foreign building concepts to Central African home builders. But like Mobutu when he says he wants a dairy, Emperors-for-Life get what they want. Thankfully, by the time I got there, the ban on traditional homes had been lifted, and virtually all new home construction was once again of the traditional design. I was there from 1982 to 1984. Bokassa had been recalled by France three years before then, and the memories of his reign were still very fresh in the minds of the villagers.

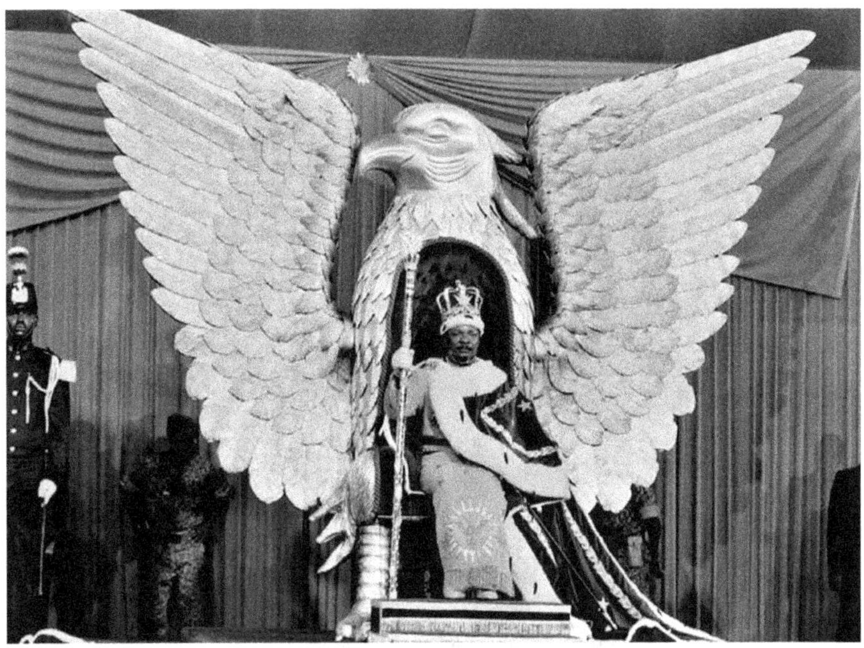

This picture says it all....

There were two methods of round hut construction. The more traditional method used a wattle wall, and the more refined method used mud bricks. To define the perimeter of the home, a stick was pounded into the ground and a string with a stick on the end etched the circle in the dirt. For a wattle home, there were vertical wooden poles, spaced about three feet apart, pounded in at the circle marked in the dirt. Smaller sticks were then woven horizontally into the posts and secured with palm-frond fibers. Clay was then mixed with straw and water to make mud for packing into the woven wattle. Once the walls were built, long poles radiated out, over the top of the walls, from a central point, where they were all affixed with fibrous cord. Purlins, the cross members that support the roofing material, were then stitched to the poles, and dried cane grass was secured to the purlins to create a thatched roof.

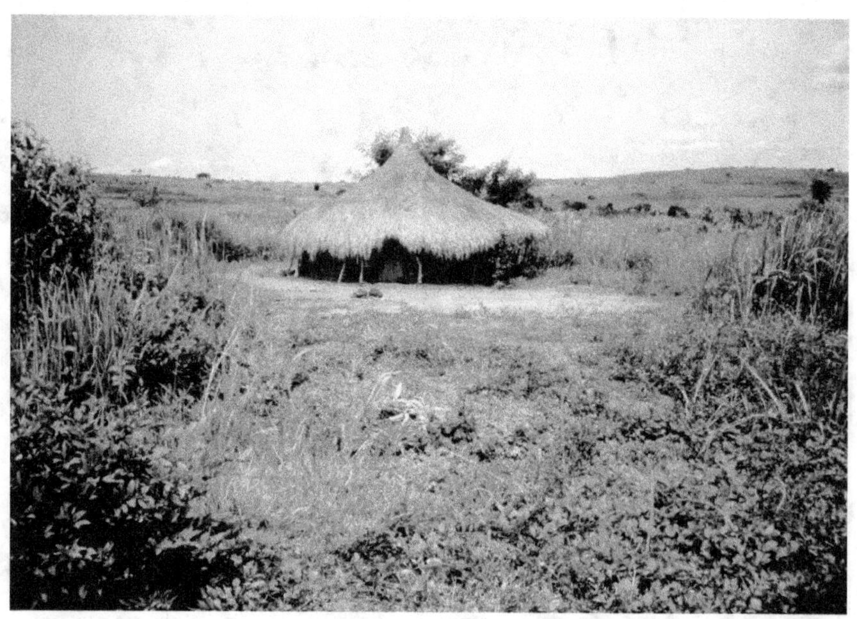

A traditional round wattle-walled house

A more expensive and labor-intensive method of construction used preformed mud bricks instead of wattle. Craftsmen who specialized in mud-brick fabrication were generally set up near a clay source. Clay was dug, mixed with some chopped straw for reinforcement, shaped into blocks, and allowed to dry in the sun. There were also wood-fired kilns where bricks were fired, but fired bricks were reserved for the wealthiest homeowners. Once the bricks were dry, they were laid out on the etched circle and the walls were built, igloo-like, using clay mortar.

Openings for windows and doors were figured into the designs, of course. Wooden planks or woven blinds then covered the openings. Because the blocks were generally not fired, they were subject to erosion from the rains. A sufficient overhang was therefore necessary to protect the vulnerable walls from erosion. Tall cane grass was cut seasonally, dried, bundled, and carried to the jobsite. Seeing this time-honored tradition of weaving a *paille* (straw) roof onto a roof frame was a thrill. Not only was this roof highly water-resistant, it was almost silent inside of the homes during a rainstorm, and much cooler than the interior of my metal-roofed house.

As the thatched roofs retained water, they began to decompose over time. When a roof began to turn to compost, it was time for a new one. Much like roofers here, there were roofers who were kept busy with reroofing projects. If the roof was sound, the rest of the house could last a long time. Here, we think having organic granola is a big deal, but in the CAR they had organic houses that were fully biodegradable. An entire house could be constructed without using a single nail.

Imagine the dismay of the home builders who were masters of a technique that had been perfected over millennia—one that resulted in a solid structure where forces were equal throughout—when they were commanded to build only rectangular houses. Now they had to figure out how to get long, straight, wobbly walls to stay up without support. They had to develop rafter ties to tie the walls to the rafters. They had to figure out how to close the gable ends and support a roof, the likes of which nobody in the villages had ever seen or built. All this because a deranged dictator thought it would make him look modern.

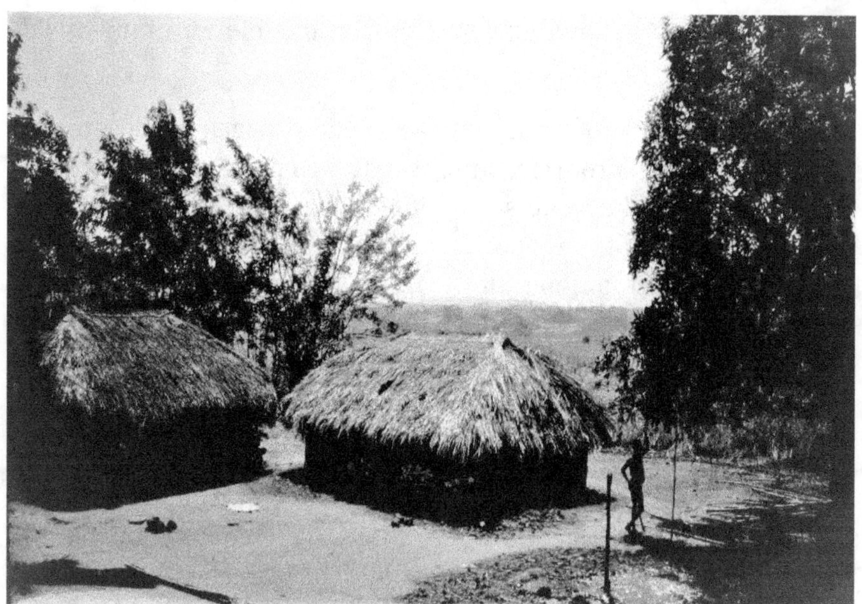

"Modern" rectangular houses

LIFE IN AN OVERDEVELOPED COUNTRY

Readjusting to the American way of life took some effort, even back in 1984. In the CAR, for example, if a piece of land was not being actively used by someone, anyone could simply claim it as theirs. When we built a fisheries station to supply fingerlings to first-time local farmers, we just built the ponds, dammed up a stream, and claimed the land as our own. There were no planning boards, zoning ordinances, property taxes, land-use permits, or environmental impact studies.

Keeping things simple is becoming more difficult, complex, and expensive every year. We have become so overdeveloped that, in some places, taking the appropriate technology approach to living is illegal. More and more, people are willingly moving to places where doing things like hanging clothes outside to dry, having a vegetable garden, keeping laying hens, cooking on a charcoal grill, or even parking a boat in the driveway will result in a fine. Thankfully, here in the north woods and in most of rural America, folks still have a healthy degree of self-reliance and are open to learning new ways to do things better, simpler, and cheaper.

My grandparents, Harry and Alma Lindgren, died in a car crash in 1973. Times were starting to change, but life on their 120-acre farm was much the same as it had been when I was toddling around on it. The current model of energy-intensive, chemical-based food production would have shocked my grandparents. The Farm Bill has become a monstrosity that tends to coddle industrial agriculture, and the USDA that administers the subsidies and rules has, due to their one-size-fits-all regulations, erected barriers for small-scale farmers wanting to grow, process, and sell their products locally. The fallout from industrial agriculture will be felt for generations. Soil erosion, the loss of soil fertility, poisons permeating our landscape, patented, gene-altered organisms, and a dead zone the size of Rhode Island in the Gulf of Mexico are some of the by-products of an industry that has been endorsed by our government. The unnatural concentration of animals in life, and in death, teeters on the brink of calamity every day. Others have written extensively on the subject, so I will just leave it at that.

Grandpa would shake his head in disbelief at where we are today, much as a Central African villager would be unable to comprehend that there are people in America who have surgery to make their stomachs smaller because we have too much food—too much unwholesome food. If I had told them that this surgery costs about as much as an automobile, they would look at me like I was telling them that we also like to vacation on the far side of the moon.

We have some real problems in America, with the health care crisis being one of the most glaring. I feel it could be greatly alleviated by doing one simple thing, and that is to *eat how our grandparents ate*. If you are in your twenties, you might have to skip back a generation and eat how your great-grandparents ate. In other words, eat whole, clean, real food grown conscientiously by local farmers. Better yet, grow as much of it as you practically can yourself. We are going to spend some time now discussing how we have applied some of what we learned from our African experience to life in America. But first, let's go to the fair.

A FAIR ASSESSMENT

Until the summer of 2011, the last time I had been to the Minnesota State Fair was in 1975, about the time I moved up to Bemidji to go to college. Prior to that time, I went to the fair every year. When I was a child, we went as a family. As I got older, one of our moms would shuttle a carload of us to the fairgrounds, dump us off, and another mom would collect us at the end of the day. As soon as the first of us got our driver's license, we were free to go whenever we wanted and stay as late as we wanted to stay. We wandered through the buildings, ate some Tom Thumb donuts and saltwater taffy, had our ten-cent glasses of ice-cold milk at the dairy booth, and usually had a hamburger and fries at the diner. Food, back then, was not all that important to us, and certainly not a reason to go to the fair. We were there mainly for the rides, and the bulk of our time was spent on the midway. Eating lots of food and going on lots of rides simply did not mix.

Our favorite ride was a huge drum that we would enter through a side door and then stand against the textured, rubber-lined wall. The drum then began turning, and once we reached sufficient rpm, the floor would drop, and centrifugal force would hold us tightly against the wall. Perhaps it was due to the blood being centrifuged to the backs of our brains, but we loved this ride. As we became more comfortable with it, we would start to show off by turning our bodies sideways, just not so far that coins fell out of our pockets. Occasionally, there was a rider who was a bit on the hefty side, so the force of gravity would exceed the centrifugal force, and they would ride down along with the floor. This person would sit on the floor, looking embarrassed, as they looked up at everyone else adhered to the wall. Sometimes there was a rider who was hovering right in the zone where gravity and centrifugal forces were in equilibrium. This person would then spend the entire ride struggling, Spider-Man-like, to remain tightly against the wall, hoping that the added force of friction would help to break the tie. There must have been a weight limit sign posted for this ride, and it must have been unpleasant for the operator to have to turn away the occasional hefty ticketholder.

I thought about this ride when our family went to the fair in the summer of 2011, and when I got there, I realized that this popular ride from my youth could not possibly still be operating. Our daughter was displaying a 4-H project, and so we all went down for the event. Returning to the state fair after thirty-six years brought back a flood of memories, but I was also overwhelmed by the changes. Thankfully the 4-H and Natural Resources buildings were as I remembered them, but almost everything else had changed. First, there were far more people, but that was to be expected. What had changed the most was that food was now king at the fair. Food vendors were everywhere, and the competition for our business was intense. It seemed to me that people were coming now first for the food, second to shop in the commercial buildings, and third to browse through the noncommercial buildings. We never even made it to the midway.

The most striking feature, however, was the size of the fairgoers. In 1975, an obese person would have stood out, and they would have been walking. In 2011, overweight people were everywhere, and many of them were atop electric scooters, which were available for rent at the entrances. These were not old folks who were too worn out to walk, and in need of assistance getting about. I saw elderly couples walking slowly, helping each other up and down curbs with stiff, worn-out joints; but they were walking. It made me wonder just how we, as a society, could have become so unfit in the past thirty-six years.

The overwhelming quantity and variety of foods available at the fair is just a microcosm of what has become available to us all, every day in America; and those who peddle this food know just how to do it. Even back in 1983, when food businesses were nowhere near as refined at enticing us with their products, I managed to gain nearly forty pounds in three months. I am not going to pretend to be an expert on diet and nutrition but, in my own experience and observations, the primary culprit is refined carbohydrates: primarily sugar, but also the refined starches.

The pancreas is, perhaps, one of our more underappreciated organs. Within it are these clusters of cells, about two grams worth, called *beta* cells. When we douse our bloodstream with lots of sugar, the beta cells sound the alarm and produce the hormone insulin to go retrieve the sugar and send it to our muscles as fuel, to our livers (where fructose is metabolized), or store the excess energy as fat. The trouble is, we are now consuming much more sugar than our clean-up crews can handle. The result is worn-out beta cells, high blood sugar levels, obesity, and type 2 diabetes. Sugar is now cleverly disguised in most of our factory-made foods.

The dozen or so food giants that now control most of the processed food industry know exactly what they are doing to get us to buy and become addicted to their products. Sugar, even when my parents were young, was relatively expensive. During the time of my great-grandparents, sugar was locked away in sugar safes by those wealthy enough to afford it, so the servants would not help themselves to it. Empires were built, and fortunes made, by controlling the sugar market. France, England, Holland, and other nations battled for centuries over the Caribbean islands, and enslaved thousands into a hellish world for sugar. Now, due to subsidies, and the use of enzymes to make sugar from the starches found in corn kernels (high-fructose corn syrup), sugar is cheap and abundant. But here I go again, pretending to be an expert. There are, fortunately, many real experts now speaking out about how sugar is wrecking our bodies. I suggest an afternoon of watching a few good TED Talks on the topic.

I can say from my personal experience that my blood sugars rise to above-normal levels when my diet includes more refined carbohydrates. If I can muster the sustained willpower to revert to a high-protein, whole-foods diet, my blood sugar levels drop significantly. Anyone who does not believe that easily digestible carbohydrates have become a major component of our American diet needs only try to avoid them for a few days.

In 2011, during the time of our visit to the state fair, Peg and I had immersed ourselves in the world of veganism. We entered this world through a well-meaning acquaintance because of health concerns. We escaped from this world nearly a year later for the same reasons. We were operating a pasty (folded meat-and-vegetable pies) shop at the time, and I saw veganism as a challenge. I created a vegan pasty, with cashew cream instead of cheese and fake butter in the crust, to add to the menu. I also came up with some recipes for spreads that were quite good. One was a paté made from chickpeas, walnuts, and my old liverwurst seasonings. It tasted amazingly like liverwurst. Even my mother was fooled by it, which was no small feat. My mother more-or-less survives on meat; or, more specifically, on fat. And salt. While she will, on occasion, consume some sweets, she has never been fond of them. If she had a small dish of ice cream, for example, it would be paired with a rolled-up piece of bologna. Mom also has squeaky-clean arteries and has weighed about the same for over sixty years. So, when she tasted my vegan spread and said, "Thank goodness you're eating meat again," I swelled with pride at my accomplishment. The dark days of veganism are brought up by our daughter at family gatherings as a bit of morbid humor. Those were the days of cashew cream, almond milk, fake butter, fake eggs, tofu, and (the one that still gives me shivers) fake cheese. Our son, Conor, had a narrow escape, having gone off to college. Sarah, however, was in middle school and trapped in a vegan household. We shamed her into eating the stuff by telling her it was for our health. But none of us could get past the fake cheese.

After nearly a year of being free from animal products, my blood work showed that my fasting blood sugars and triglyceride levels were at an all-time high. A vegan diet, unless one is very regimented about food choices, is, by default, a high-carbohydrate diet. Peg, meanwhile, had begun sneaking eggs into her diet, and our vegan world was starting to crumble. About this time, I heard a radio interview with Gary Taubes about his book, *Why We Get Fat*. This was the first I had heard about metabolic syndrome, insulin resistance, and how our bodies convert carbohydrates to fats. It all intuitively made sense to me. Sarah received a shock when she came up one morning for her tofu scrambler and was met, instead, with a platter of bacon and eggs (without bread). Her response was, "I'm stuck in a family of bipolar eaters!" And then she ate all of her bacon.

Following several months of eating a high-protein (and high-fat) diet, I went in for an extensive work-up for a new life insurance policy. The blood work showed my blood sugars down by twenty-five percent, and all other levels also in the lower-than-average categories. The results were so good, in fact, that I was given an additional fifteen percent premium discount. I was good at following a low-carbohydrate diet at first, and my weight stayed at high school levels. I was eating my burgers without the bun, ordering salads when dining out, and eating only peanuts as a snack. Slowly, however, carbohydrates began to creep, insidiously, into my diet. The buns returned, the beer, the pasta, and the bread, and the *we're on vacation so one ice cream cone won't hurt* type of rationalizations became more frequent.

It is just plain hard, in our society, to curtail the consumption of refined carbohydrates. As I write this, it is the mid-January, post-holidays, too-cold-for-outdoor-exercise time of year, and I have ten extra pounds to show for it. I find that, initially, the problem is abated by simply avoiding the bathroom scale. Eventually, though, I am forced to look down and see myself in that one photo, and that's it; it's time to get serious and climb onto the scale for an initial assessment. The numbers that show up are just the incentive I need to take command of the situation.

I know it can be done. I just need to make a *shift* in my diet, not go on a diet. When the annual trip to see family members in southwest Florida draws near and the thought of that one picture re-emerges, I can curtail the carbs and drop eight pounds in about two weeks. The picture I am referring to is the one of me on the beach in the Bahamas, back in the pre-vegan days, when an impressive bowl of ice cream accompanied every Twins game (which was just about every night). In this picture, I had just ridden in on the surf, and was rocking on my belly, pretending to be a beached whale, while Sarah took the picture. The problem was that my re-enactment left little to the imagination; I looked like a beluga in swim trunks. As I write this, I have just stepped onto the scale for the first time this year, and the numbers have shocked me into action. I fried up two of our own eggs for breakfast, skipped the toast, and I am going to have to break it to Peg and Sarah tonight that the pasta dishes will not be on the menu for a while. I'm going to town to buy a nice ham instead. You see, there is this trip to Florida coming up in a month...

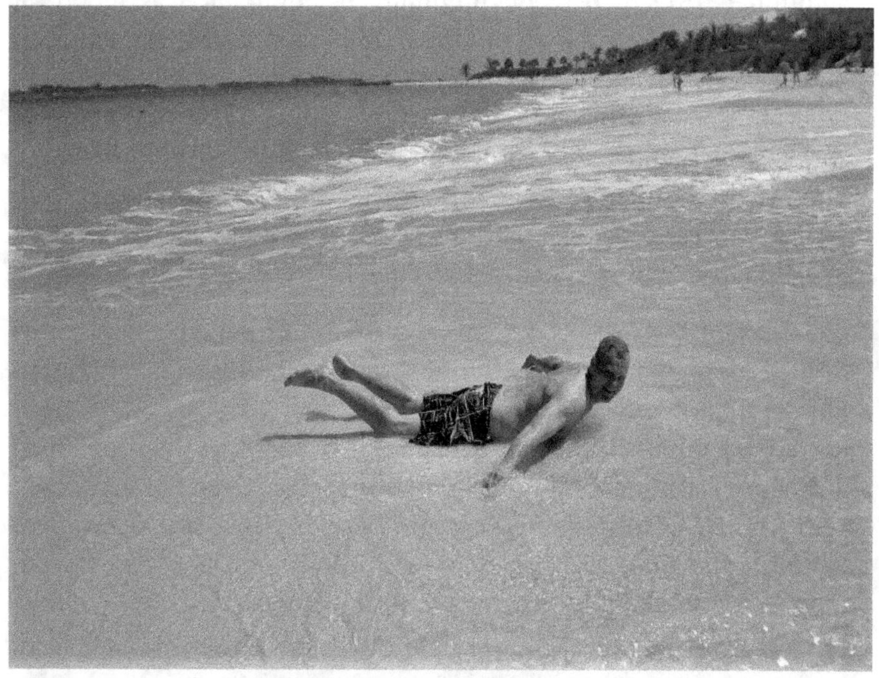

Again, a picture says it all....

DEFERRED AWARENESS

If there was to be a committee formed to design a monument to the unprecedented wastefulness of our modern society, they could not come up with one more appropriate than a cruise ship. My mother, to celebrate her eightieth birthday, took all eighteen (now there are twenty-one) members of her family on a cruise from Miami to Nassau, Bahamas. This was in 2010, and it was on this trip that the action-stimulating photograph of me was taken on the beach. We had never been on a cruise and having the entire family together in such a setting was, of course, wonderful. As anyone who has lived in a third-world country can attest, however, that experience becomes etched into your soul. There was to be no carefree cruising for me.

I simply could not ignore the sight of families, after their meal, pushing their chairs back from a table that was left heaping-full of uneaten food. There was food everywhere, in endless supply, twenty-four hours a day. I had become acclimated to displays of wastefulness and gluttony after returning from the CAR, but never on such a grand scale; and far too many of the passengers (including myself) qualified to receive the *bien engraissé* compliment. Our ship had to have discarded a ton of food every day, and it did not help matters knowing that this floating resort was being shoved through the water with a fuel economy that was measured in *feet* per gallon. I have read that, in the past, this wasted food was simply ground up and disposed of in the ocean once the ships were in international waters. I could only hope that there is now at least enough oversight over these floating resorts to require that the waste be returned to port and disposed of in an approved facility. But what is *approved* is not something most of us care to even think about. I call it *deferred awareness* (like what I am doing when I avoid stepping on the bathroom scale).

We all, at some point, have enjoyed the feeling of looking down on others from what we perceive as the moral high ground. The aware shopper who comes to the supermarket carrying their reusable, recycled-plastic shopping bag can watch disapprovingly as the rest of us have our items bagged into those environment-destroying plastic bags. What the reusable shopping bag shopper would just as soon not be made aware of, however, is that one quarter of the food that they are carrying home in their *green* bags will likely be wasted. They also would prefer not knowing that there are dumpsters full of outdated, blemished, poorly selling, or spoiled food being carted off from the back of their favorite supermarket every day.

More than forty percent of the food grown and shipped at great expense to supermarkets, restaurants, and our homes, is wasted. About sixty percent of that wasted food is buried in landfills. The other forty percent is incinerated. When food is buried in a landfill, it undergoes anaerobic decomposition, which produces methane gas. Methane is a greenhouse gas that is something like twenty times more potent than carbon dioxide. Since food is mostly water, trying to get it to burn in an incinerator requires an awful lot of energy. Just try burning a box full of overripe bananas sometime. Once it does burn, there is all that ash to deal with, which ends up in (you guessed it) the landfill.

The average household wastes twenty-five percent of its food, which is like tossing $1,000 or more into the trash. So why, at a time when we are so aware of *green* activities, like recycling paper and containers, do we turn a blind eye to the most wasteful, expensive, and environmentally dangerous practice of all, and one that we are all actively participating in? Mainly, it's because it is so easy to do, and it is done so insidiously. If most of us saw what was being trucked away from the backs of our supermarkets, we would be shocked. But we will never see it. This part of the operation will never be part of a tour. Our municipalities are never going to print the tonnage of food waste carted to the landfill, or the tipping fees that were collected in the process. We will never see it, and we will never hear about it.

So, what can we do about it? Some surplus food makes its way to food shelves and soup kitchens. Due to the many constraints, such as regulations, store policies, the fear of lawsuits, and transportation costs, this is a small percentage of the total amount of wasted food. Changing our habits would certainly go a long way toward reducing the amount of food wasted in our homes. Joel Salatin, in his top-notch book, *Folks, This Ain't Normal*, argues that all this food waste should be fed to chickens and pigs. Sure, let's do that wherever it is most feasible. But I think the best solution is a municipality-wide composting operation. Rather than feeding folks foods that are high in refined carbohydrates, I say we should turn those glazed donuts into rich compost, and then use this composted material to grow nutritious leafy greens. The technology is out there for large-scale composting. Some cities have been doing it for years. I am not advocating another unfunded government mandate. Municipal composting simply is the smart thing to do, both from an environmental and an economic perspective.

After living in the CAR, the thought of throwing food scraps in the trash is just plain wrong. Nothing went to waste in Africa. Even a discarded sardine can became a pull-toy for a child, who would fashion wooden axles and wheels, attach a cord, and pull the little car around the clean-swept yard. When I was new to my post in Bangassou, I recall meeting with some aspiring fish farmers under a *paillote* in a village. This thatch-roofed structure provides valuable shade and serves as a central meeting-place in the village; it's a community center of sorts. There were, as always, some children on the periphery, observing and learning from the adults. I thought I would impress these children with my cleverness, so I tore a piece of paper from my notebook, folded it into a sleek paper airplane, and sent my creation soaring across the paillote. As it skidded to a stop in the dust, I was expecting excited chatter, but was met instead with a puzzling silence. One of the older boys then walked over to my creation, picked it up, brought it to a bench, and began to carefully, almost reverently, unfold and flatten it, in an attempt to return it to its original shape as a piece of unused notebook paper.

 I will never forget the look of disgust I got from that boy. I was the important white patron who had arrived on a motorcycle, which was on par with someone here showing up at a party in a helicopter. I was supposed to be held in awe, not contempt. As an American, I never gave a thought to a piece of notebook paper as something having value. But to these children, a notebook was a treasure, and a new, unused piece of paper would never be turned into a toy, not before it had been written on, on both sides and in the margins, and it had served its purpose. It could then be used to fashion a cone for vending peanuts in the market. This boy had taught me an early lesson, and I was to learn many more from those who were much wiser than I was.

We take so much for granted in America, where we are so distanced from shortages. In the CAR, a bent nail would never be thrown away. A bent nail here is something to be discarded, especially on a jobsite, where it would cost more to have a worker take the time to straighten a nail than to simply grab a new one. In the CAR, a nail would be a valuable possession. To run out of nails for a project would mean setting the project aside for perhaps several weeks until more nails arrived from Bangui, if they could afford more nails in the first place. The way we waste our resources, it is little wonder that the rest of the world looks at us the way the boy in the paillote looked at me.

I grew up with Depression-era parents. My mother was born in 1930 and was somewhat insulated from the deprivation of those times, having grown up on the rich prairie farmland northwest of Willmar. My mother did not have electricity until the late 1940s, and my grandparents were certainly not living in great comfort, but they also never went hungry. My father, however, was born in 1923, and grew up on the sandy woodlands northwest of Park Rapids, just south of Bemidji. It was the lure of cheap land that got my grandfather to move his family north after losing his farm in Iowa in the 1920s. So, he packed his family and all their worldly goods into a Model T Ford truck and brought them to a little town called Two Inlets. He could not glean a living from this land, however, and had to forfeit it. He then bought another farm a few miles closer to the town of Osage, where he and my grandmother raised their six children.

My dad told many stories about growing up on these farms. Despite their obvious poverty, his tales were mostly told without regret. He fondly told tales of hunting prairie chickens or catching bluegills to provide for the family. He told of how thick the ice was on the insides of the windows in the farmhouse in the winter, and how he would rise early to get a fire started in the woodstove. He recalled the names of all their dogs and horses, and how Grandpa would plug away, an acre at a time, clearing trees from the land to put more sandy soil into production. Dad was a hard worker and had been one by necessity since the time he was a young boy. He certainly had reason enough to be bitter, but bitterness never surfaced in the stories of his youth.

I have read many books about World War II, from D-Day to the Philippines—where my father served—and the authors refer to these young men as the Greatest Generation. My dad was one of them, and most of them came from similar Depression-era backgrounds. They came from places where they had to work hard to survive, and they had no expectations of anyone. They were grateful for what they had, and they did not covet. They were content.

My dad received the Bronze Star from President Truman for his role in the Battle of Luzon in the Philippines. He spent more than 160 days in combat, sleeping in foxholes and under tanks. He was a Technical Sergeant who drove a tank along mountain trails at night with no lights. He survived a tank exploding while he was underneath it. When he died at seventy-two from ALS, he still had shrapnel embedded in his skull. I did not even know that my dad had received the Bronze Star until the last year of his life.

These were the men who became the fathers to us kids on our safe, secure suburban blocks. These are the fathers who told us not to waste the food on our plates, or waste energy or water taking luxurious showers. These are the fathers who, unfortunately, were seen by us kids as out-of-touch relics who could not adapt to modern times of plenty. So, when I would stomp on the floor above one of my own showering children, as a gentle reminder that four minutes was way too long, I also established myself as a meddling, out-of-touch relic.

The last members of the Greatest Generation are now dying away, and with their passing we are losing much of their spirit of gratefulness. With gratitude came humility, and with that came a great nation.

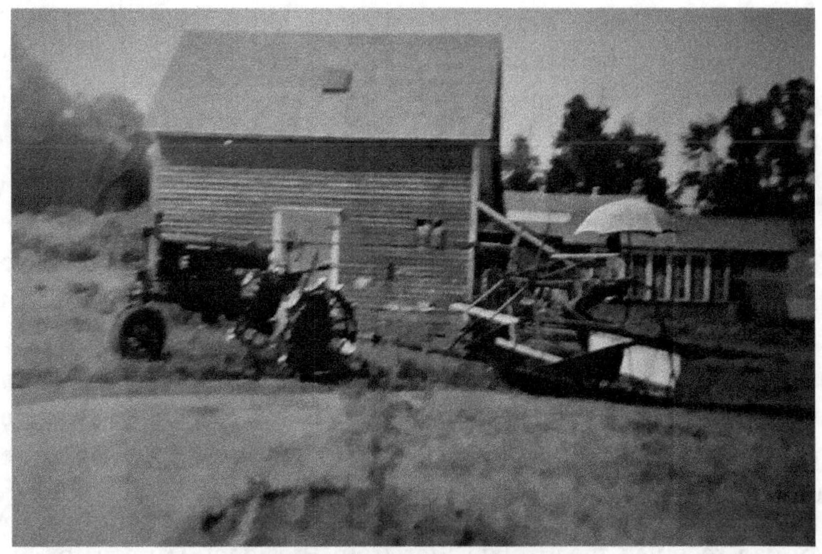

My mother's farm when she was young

COMPOSTING 101

Composting in the CAR was somewhat of a foreign concept, partly because having wasted food was a foreign concept. Any food scraps were found by the always-hungry pigs. As we previously discussed, livestock was not fed, and they therefore had to fend for themselves. The Sango word for animal is *niama*. The word for meat is also *niama*. As the name implies, the fate of an animal in the CAR is well-ordained. Peg once tried to assign a human name to a chicken that belonged to the family she lived with. She was informed that this was not done. One does not name their meat. Fish were also niama and feeding them was as foreign to the villagers as feeding (or naming) a chicken. Why would they toss edible greens into the ponds for the fish to eat, when those greens could go into a sauce to feed the family?

Fortunately, the species of tilapia best suited for pond culture, *Tilapia nilotica*, was not only fast growing, capable of reproduction every six weeks, and tolerant of very low oxygen levels, but it was also able to thrive by filtering phytoplankton (algae) from the water. To promote a good phytoplankton bloom, the pond water must contain nutrients. Those nutrients came from organic material composted in bins that were installed in the ponds. Before we jump into the compost bins, though, I want to expand a bit on one other remarkable adaptation of *Tilapia nilotica*.

Being a cichlid, tilapia are nest builders. The pond bottoms were a lunar landscape of excavated bowl-shaped nests made by the much larger, strikingly colorful males. The females would deposit their eggs in the nests, and the males would then fertilize them. Once fertilized, the female would scoop up the eggs in her mouth, where they would remain until they hatched, in about twelve days. This is where the ability to filter plankton through her gills to feed herself became an important asset; it is tough to eat otherwise with a mouth full of kids. This mouth brooding adaptation keeps the fertilized eggs safe from predators. Even after the eggs hatched, if danger threatened, a mom could call all the kids back into her gaping mouth to keep them safe. It was a thrill to watch dozens of tiny fry scoot into and out of mom's open mouth. This could not continue long, of course, since it soon became cramped quarters. But what a mom!

To fertilize the ponds, we built semicircular compost bins from woven sticks. Since the debris that was going into the bins was not usable food, the farmers soon learned to keep the bins filled with fallen palm fronds, rotted paille from a reroofing project, or any vegetative matter for which they had no other use. It was mostly carbon-based material, but in the tropical heat it released enough nitrogen, phosphorus, and potassium to promote an algal bloom. The best materials were the ones that required a truck, which was one of my justifications for having one so often. If I had a truck to haul them to the site, I could obtain cotton seed and coffee hulls, by-products from the French-run processing facilities, for free. I mostly restricted the use of this better material for our fingerling production station, since it did farmers little good to learn a technique that required the use of a truck.

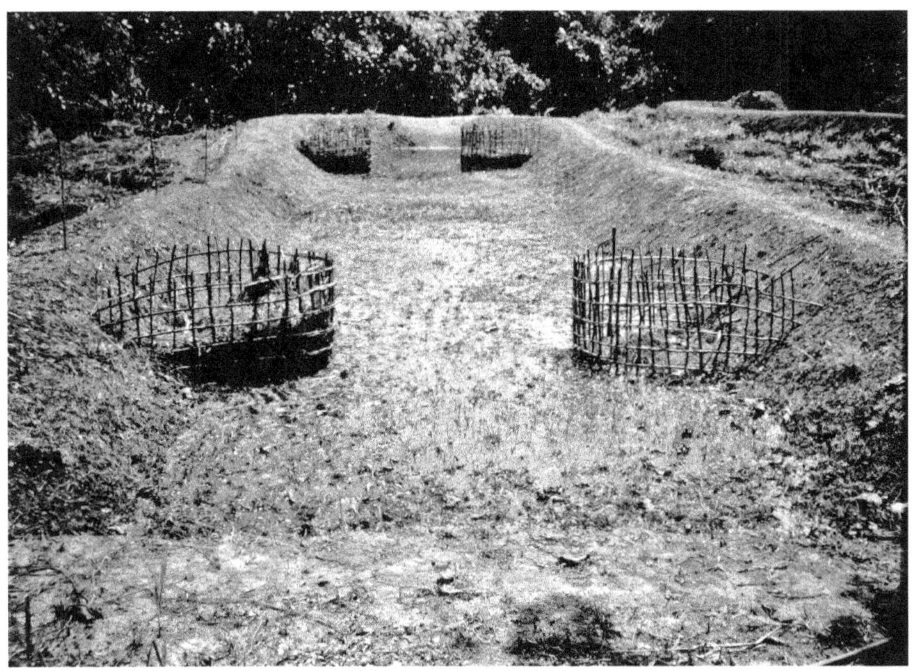

Compost bins in a new pond at Oyé Carrefour

LEAVES: THE SECRET TO SUCCESS

We have learned a secret from our forests, and it is this: *All any plant needs to thrive for an entire growing season is a two-inch deep layer of rich humus*. Humus is the rich organic layer found under the leaf litter on the forest floor. It consists almost entirely of decomposed leaves that break down slowly in the cool, moist, oxygen-poor environment under the insulating leaf litter. The primary decomposers for this job are fungi and invertebrates (worms and insects). Trees are never in a hurry. If it takes a season or two for a layer of leaves to decompose, so be it. With the only inputs being air, water, and sunlight, a forest can thrive for thousands of years. That, at a time when the word is so overused and abused, is the true meaning of *sustainable*.

Since we lack the patience and longevity of trees, we want our compost in weeks, not years. To accomplish this, we hire aerobic bacteria to do the job. They work very fast, but they have some fairly strict job requirements. Their food supply needs to have about thirty parts carbon to each part nitrogen. They also need air, moisture, and warmth. Without going into the specifics of composting, I want to at least give you the fundamentals and leave the method, whether to use a rotating composter, static pile, or bin, up to you.

To speed up the process, we must first increase the surface area of the leaves. We do this by using a lawn mower. For small jobs, we choose our self-propelled walk-behind mulching lawn mower with a rear bagging system. For the main cleanup, we first chop and windrow the leaves using our riding mower, and then come along with a large-capacity lawn sweeper to claim the chopped leaves. Why we did not buy an inexpensive lawn sweeper years ago is a question we get from our children, who were not especially fond of raking leaves. But those were the Dark Ages, before we understood the value of using our leaves for gardening.

Once we have our carbon supply (chopped leaves), we add nitrogen. The 30:1 ratio of carbon to nitrogen preferred by bacteria is attained by mixing up a 3:1 ratio of browns to greens. Confused? This is usually where we lose folks, by saying 30:1 and then, in the same breath, saying 3:1. So which is it?

Material is considered *brown* if it has a carbon (cellulose) to nitrogen (protein) ratio of greater than 30:1. All plant material contains more cellulose than it does protein. Cellulose is the carbohydrate that forms the fibers that give plants structure. Without cellulose, plants could not stand up. Unlike animals, which rely on proteins to build muscle, plants bulk up simply by standing in the sun, turning air, sunlight and water into cellulose. I am always amazed to see a massive, towering white pine in our woods and know that this majestic tree was made mostly from air and water.

Leaves have a carbon to nitrogen ratio of about 200:1, so they are called a *brown* material. Coffee grounds, our favorite *green* material, has a carbon to nitrogen ratio of about 20:1. This, of course, simply adds to the confusion, because coffee grounds are definitely brown, but are still considered a green material. Coffee grounds, however, are the roasted, ground-up seeds from the coffee plant, and seeds are the storehouses for the amino acids that make up the DNA that replicates more coffee plants.

Fresh green grass clippings are also about 20:1, and are another excellent source of nitrogen. This explains why bison, cattle, and horses can grow to become massively muscled creatures while consuming (almost nonstop) little besides green vegetation. To achieve an approximate 30:1 ratio in our compost material, we simply add about three parts brown to one part green material. For example, for every five-gallon bucket of coffee grounds, green grass clippings, or kitchen scraps added to the compost bin, we would add *three* five-gallon buckets full of chopped leaves, sawdust, or wood chips.

Obtaining a five-gallon bucket full of coffee grounds on our own is a tall order. Even I don't drink that much coffee. Coffee grounds, however, are such a rich nitrogen source that it is worth visiting an accommodating local coffee shop and leaving them a clean bucket to fill with grounds. Besides being a good nitrogen source, they are also rich in calcium, phosphorus, potassium, magnesium, and copper, while also improving soil tilth and structure. Unlike the coffee that is brewed from them, coffee grounds themselves are not acidic.

Next, we add oxygen, and to do this we tumble our mixture. Some of our compost tumblers turn automatically using a windshield wiper motor, bicycle sprockets, and a serpentine belt from a car. This is an invention that I am sure Central Africans would get a kick out of. Anyone interested in constructing such a composter can contact us; we are happy to share ideas. A simpler, but less fun, method is to turn the material by hand, either in a rotating drum or in a static pile or bin. The problem with a compost bin here in northern Minnesota is that it is just a frozen block of material for six months or more. We have dug into our static piles well into June, to find cores of still-frozen material.

To keep the process going, the material must also be moist but not sopping wet. Every book on composting you will ever read uses the wrung-out sponge analogy. If liquid is running from the drum or bin, add more carbon, such as sawdust, to sop it up. If it is too dry, add more water. If there is an ammonia odor, there is too much nitrogen, so add more carbon. If it is not heating up, and there is enough oxygen and moisture, add more nitrogen. Adding a bucketful of fresh grass clippings will get my glasses to steam up when I open the composter the next morning. Like properly operating a woodstove, being a compost manager becomes somewhat of an art.

Composting is fun and it feels good to know that virtually no organic matter leaves our property or makes its way to the landfill. The material that is unfit for our composters goes to what we call the feel-good pile. This a static pile that receives the avocado skins and pits, orange peels, and any of the large, woody items that would still resemble themselves after spending six weeks in the composter. Animal products do not generally go into the composters or onto the feel-good pile due to the formation of the breakdown proteins associated with their decomposition. With names like *putrescine* and *cadaverine*, these breakdown proteins live up to their names. Perhaps someday we will have a composter large enough to handle these materials.

When we process twenty-five chickens, we produce plenty of waste, which we bury in a former garden plot. To do this I use a very handy machine, an earth auger attachment for my ice auger powerhead. It is a simple matter to drill a few thirty-inch-deep holes and bury the waste products. I do the same for fish guts. After cleaning fish, out comes the auger, and they are soon well beyond the reach of any marauding skunks. After nearly twenty years of burying fish and chicken parts in one area of our yard, we now have some very happy honeyberry bushes growing there.

I LOVE TO MESS WITH WATER

Like many Minnesotans, I love water, even if it exists as a solid for half the year. When I was a kid, there were few projects more enjoyable for me than constructing a series of dams on the stream course that appeared along the curb on our street following a rain, or resulting from the neighbor's poorly placed lawn sprinkler. As an adult, I had the unique opportunity to do much the same thing in the CAR.

A suitable pond site was one where a small stream—generally one I could leap across—flowed down a valley with gentle grassy slopes, at least on one side. The ponds we built were called *diversion ponds* because we were diverting water from the stream and directing this water through a diversion canal above the ponds to fill them. These were some of the most enjoyable projects I have ever been involved with, but they were some of the most baffling for the fish farmers. Nobody, in their experience, had ever taken water out of a streambed and brought it fifty feet up the hillside. They always began with skepticism and (I imagine) some hilarious stories around the evening fires at the start of the project about how the patron thought he could get water to run uphill.

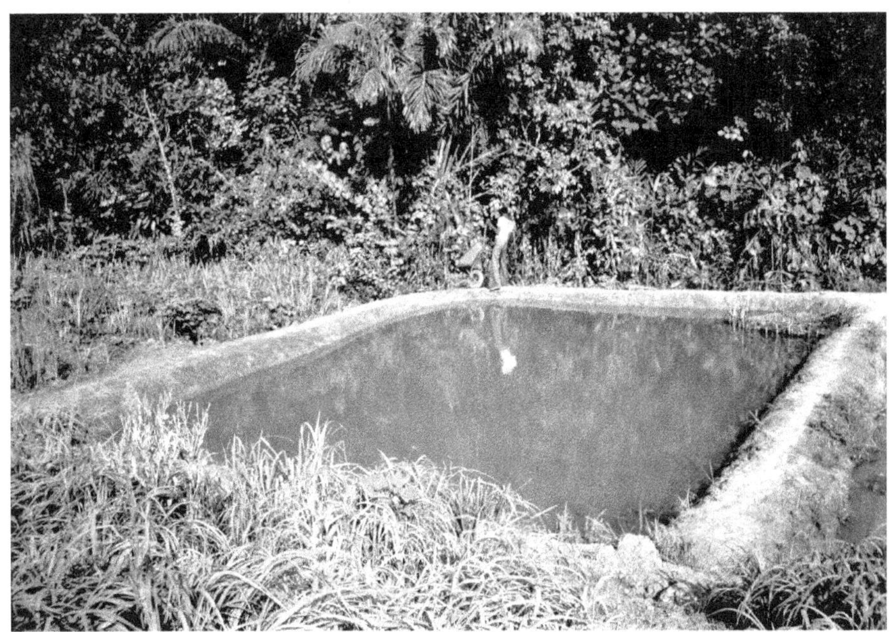

Diversion pond being filled for the first time in Damba-just a bit of dike work remaining

To understand diversion ponds, we must first understand that the reason the water flowed in the stream was because the valley floor sloped downward. All that was needed to survey the canal route was a simple hand-level and two sticks of equal height. If I were to stand at the upper end of the valley with my hand-level poised on top of a stick that was placed in the streambed, and my assistant walked one hundred feet downstream and stood his stick up in the streambed, my hand-level would shoot well over the top of his stick. This would prove that the streambed sloped downward which, of course, is why the water was flowing. Here is where I lost my farmers; I would stay at my spot, but my assistant would walk up the slope with his stick until the hand-level showed that the tops of our two sticks were at the same elevation. This would eventually place him a good distance uphill from the streambed— far enough uphill to fit in some fishponds. We would find this level along the hillside where our two sticks were at the same elevation, and stake it out as our canal route. Using picks, shovels, and wheelbarrows, a one-foot-wide and one-foot-deep trench was dug, with the removed material brought down in wheelbarrows to be added to the pond dikes.

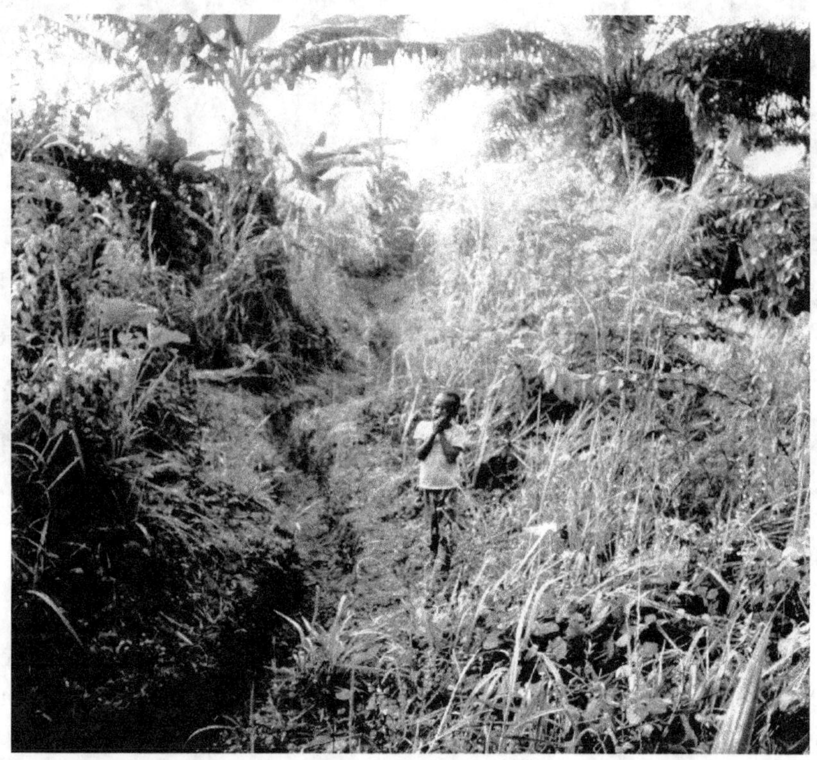

A diversion canal at Damba, following the contours of the terrain

I hope I have not lost anyone here, since it is much easier to show than it is to explain. As the canal was being dug, sometimes through hard, laterite rock, the farmers would say, "We are willing to do this work because you are the patron, but we would like to point out that water cannot run uphill." It certainly looked that way. Once we were past the area where we were going to build the ponds, we would simply divert the water back down to the streambed. So, it was always fun, once the canal was completed, to break open the earthen plug separating the stream from the canal and watch the water begin to flow into it. At first, it was not too impressive, as the dry ground sucked up most of the water. Once the soil was saturated, however, the water began flowing along its length, followed by a bunch of excitedly chattering grown men who had just witnessed the patron directing water to run uphill.

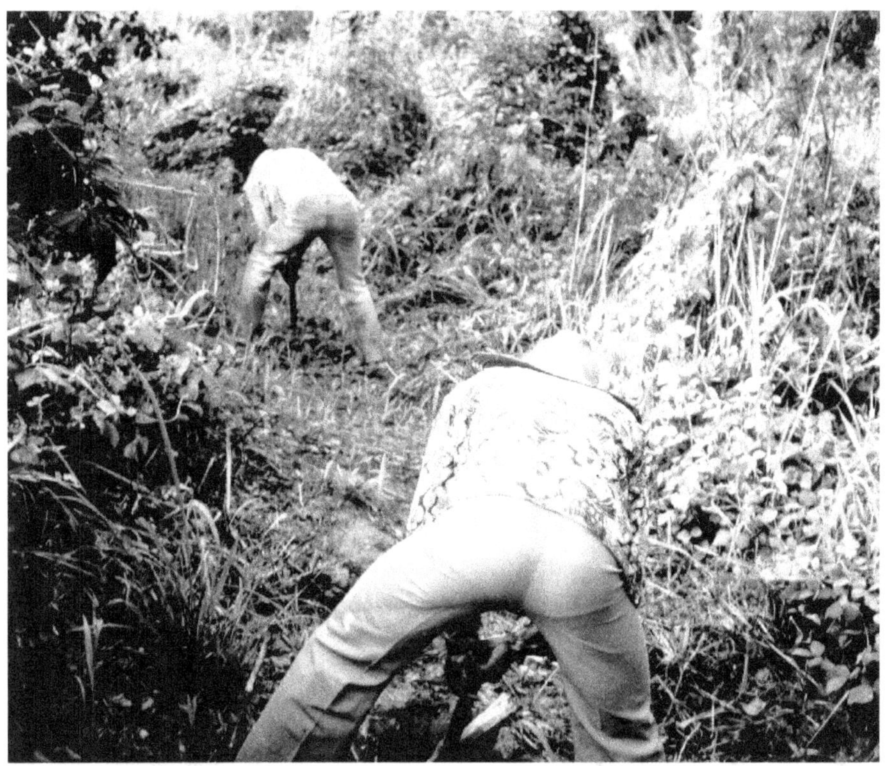

Digging canals was hard work that required a leap of faith

The ponds were constructed using what we called the cut-and-fill method. The bottom of the pond, adjacent to the stream, was basically at ground level, and dikes were built up to hold the water. As we went uphill, we cut into the hillside to maintain a level pond bottom and hauled this excavated material down to build the lower dikes. It was hard labor, and none of these farmers were being paid to do it. This was an act of faith, which is why I had them build the canal before starting on the ponds. Once there was water flowing through a canal, well above the pond construction site, they saw that this idea was not so crazy after all. But it was hard work nonetheless. First, the sod layer had to be removed from the footprint of the pond, otherwise water would seep under the dikes and the ponds would leak. The clay content was generally high enough to create leakproof dikes, but they required relentless tamping during their construction to compact the soil. We had a tamper, but those Irish Setter boots of mine were considered the best tampers of all. I was therefore elected to stomp down on each added wheelbarrow-load of soil.

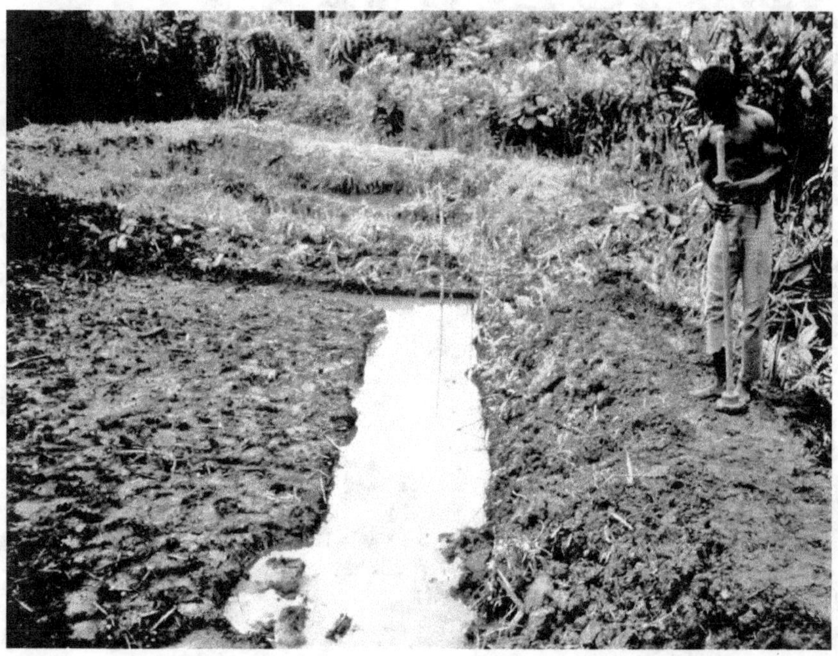

Sod is removed, then complete root system removal where the dikes will go-all done by hand.

One of my favorite places on earth was the fisheries station my three agents and I built at a place called Oye´ Carrefour. Unlike the ideal pond site, this was a fairly flat, grassy field bordered by a small stream. Since there was insufficient elevation change for a diversion canal above the ponds, we had to dam the stream and fill the ponds from the reservoir behind the dam. We had been taught in Oklahoma how to build concrete control structures called *monks* (I have no idea why they are called that) that used removable wooden slats to control the water level. Since this was to be a station to supply fingerlings for first-time farmers, I decided it was worth the time and expense to do it right by building a permanent control structure, as well as a concrete box-culvert for the water to pass under the earthen dam. We also had a blast building it.

I needed the use of a truck, of course, and I just happened to have one at my disposal. So, I ordered bags of cement from Zaire, which came over by pirogue. We dug a truckload of beach sand from a dry-season sandbar along the river, and hauled it, and the cement, up to the job site. I somehow managed to obtain the lumber for the forms, and the rebar from Zaire. The gravel was sifted, by hand, from the streambed at the jobsite. I kick myself for leaving it behind, but I found a Stone-Age tool while we were sifting gravel. When I showed it to my agents, they verified that it was a tool from *les anciens*, the ancient folks. The grooves and notches, where the head had attached to a handle, were obvious— even to me. I brought it back to Mobaye, but I do not recall what became of it. I will never know now, but I may have briefly held in my hand the head of a tool that had once been used as part of some 10,000-year-old appropriate technology project.

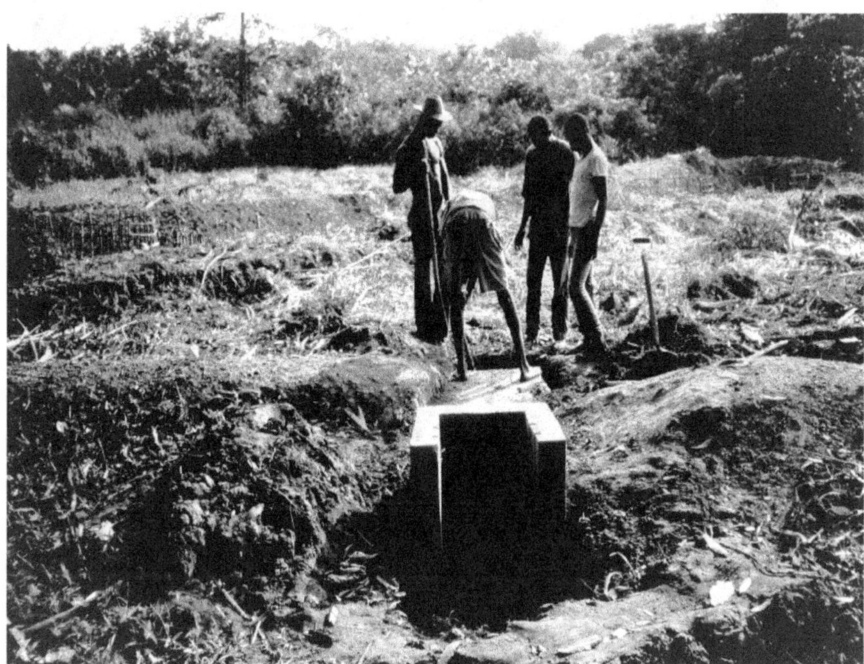

The monk and concrete box culvert under construction

There was, unfortunately, a large mango tree that was situated right in the middle of our reservoir. So, when the boards were in place and the reservoir was filled, water came three feet up the trunk of the tree. We speculated about whether-or-not the flooding would kill the tree. Since the boards were only in place when we needed to add water to the ponds, I guessed that the tree would survive, and it did not show any signs of stress while I was there. Sitting on the dike under the shade of this majestic tree, hearing water trickle over the top boards as it flowed through our concrete culvert under the dike, was part of what made this such a magical place. It filled us all with pride to look over the handsome ponds that had been hand-built and were teeming with tilapia. It was also fun to see our reservoir being enjoyed by other villagers. One farmer started a banana plantation that was irrigated with water from our reservoir.

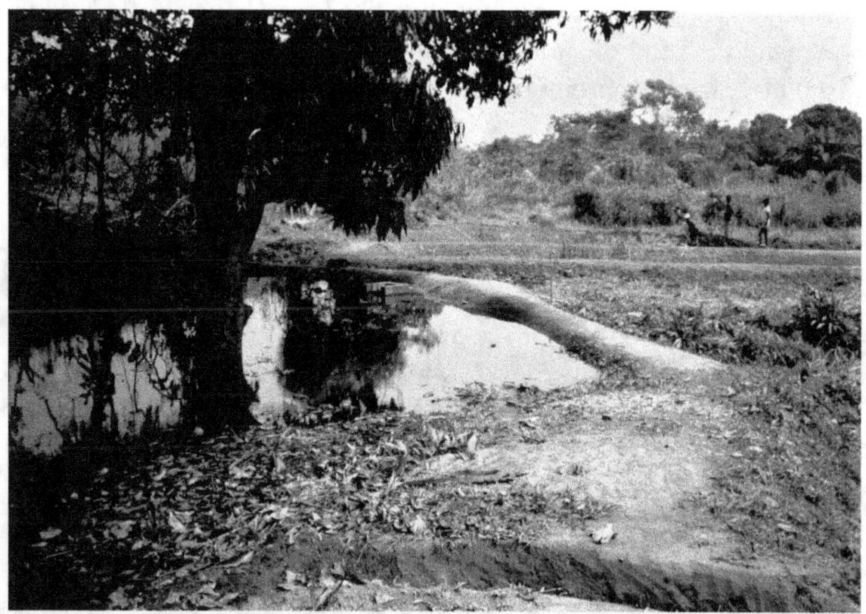

Completed dam with the flooded mango tree. Ponds being built in the background

The CAR is such a sad place now, with so much violence and danger. I can only hope that the ponds are still filled with fish, and that the dam is still supplying life-giving water to crops. One thing is certain: Our concrete monk will still be there 1,000 years from now.

The CAR had such potential, which makes its current situation such a tragedy. There was a considerable amount of petty theft when we were there. I know of no volunteer who escaped being robbed. In Mobaye, it was all blamed on the folks from Zaire, of course. But we never felt unsafe. It was a time of innocence that has now been shattered by violence, hatred, and fear. The Peace Corps, as of this writing, has pulled out of the CAR, due to its unstable and downright dangerous conditions.

I thought about it then and I think about it now, that the CAR was blessed with some of the best farmers and farmland in the world. All they needed from their government were decent roads and a means to get their crops to a market. Given half a chance, these farmers could feed their whole nation, and perhaps much of Africa. It would have helped, of course, if there had also been a health care system to control diseases like malaria and the whole host of other parasites. It seemed so simple to provide decent roads and health care, and let the villagers transform the CAR into the jewel of Central Africa. Why must the pattern of self-serving dictatorships repeat itself over and over throughout so much of Africa? I believed then, and still believe, that the CAR should be led by a strong woman from a village. She would, of course, need the strength and determination to resist the destructive temptations that come with power, but if she ran the country like the women ran the villages, great things could be accomplished.

Following that brief tirade, I intended to just leave it at that. I really want to avoid the pitfall of becoming too preachy. But then my sister and brother-in-law went and downsized their home. This meant decluttering, which meant jettisoning all those sentimental keepsakes that start looking an awful lot like clutter. So, she sent me a bundle of letters that I had sent to them while I was in the CAR. This was just too good of an opportunity to pass up. Here were firsthand accounts of what the younger me saw happening in the CAR at the time. So here we go, back to Mobaye on May 19, 1984:

...I'm real proud of the work I have accomplished in these areas. I feel good about the survival of fish culture after the aid is pulled out. The only way a project will be successful is if the idea being presented is one that is feasible and practical here in Africa... I've become very critical of aid programs...It is true that many food aid programs are not only very expensive, but do more harm than good. Since January I have fed close to 30 sacks of American corn meal to the fish. I'm raising corn-fed tilapia over here, compliments of the World Food Program. The stuff becomes inedible in a very short time because of bugs. So I feed it to the fish. At a cost of $50 a sack? People can grow corn here. They can grow anything here. This country can feed all of Africa. But handouts destroy any market that might exist. Japan gave the poor starving people here (I think that was sarcasm) *tons of rice and as a result, rice farmers could hardly give their crops away...Very little of the food ever reaches the people. It is sold by government officials, and the food that does reach the people is probably sold in the markets, like it is here, to buy food they like. To exist, these countries—even the poorest ones—must become self-sufficient. Handouts hinder their efforts. The only thing limiting food production is a market. The old colonial powers are also to blame. France has as much control over CAR now as they did 30 years ago, probably more. What is happening now is that France is threatening to reduce aid if CAR cannot start to balance the trade deficit. A French company takes cotton out of CAR. So the government went around to every village and made it mandatory for everyone to have a cotton field. If they are caught on the roads in the morning, they are questioned and made to go back to their fields. Each village has a quota they must meet. Now, when I go to work the only people in the villages are the very old and the very young people. If they are working for me that is a good excuse, so I can still find people to build ponds. But it's colonialism through a puppet government. Cotton is an awful lot of work to raise here. It robs nutrients from the soil and has very little return. One of my*

agents made 10,000CFA in 2 years raising cotton. That's $25. They can make 50,000CFA in 3 months raising corn on the same field. Or 110,000CFA in one year with 3 fishponds. Peanuts, manioc and rice are other food crops that can be raised for a fair profit. Instead they must raise cotton at gun-point. It makes me mad. My opinion of France is pretty low right now.

These are just my thoughts after living on the village level here for a while. I say keep the free food in the States, and help Africans grow their own. But that doesn't mean to send over tractors either. Africa is littered with broken down John Deeres. An appropriate contribution would be to send someone over to live at the village level and teach the techniques of animal traction, for plowing and transport. Or teaching other forms of appropriate technology—I like that word. Well, that's enough of that...

It most certainly is. My poor sister. My brother-in law, Dell, is a now-retired pastor. They were serving a church in Iowa at the time. I seem to recall that they had innocently inquired in a previous letter about what churches could do to help the poor people in Africa. It must have been a rainy day, because they certainly got an earful. Aside from the excessive use of *italics*, it really is interesting (I think) to hear exactly what I thought about the situation thirty-five years ago. Now back to ponds.

Some of the great things that I would dream of as I explored the breathtaking rolling savanna in my district were great big dams across large ravines to create hillside ponds. These ponds of my dreams were not our handmade fishponds. These would be *barrage* ponds that would require heavy equipment for their construction. During the rainy season, the skies would open up every day and rain would come down in torrents. It would rain so hard that the roads often became impassable. Rain barriers were set up to keep vehicles from using the roads when they became more like rivers.

The terrain I worked in was dotted with ravines that were ideal for the construction of hillside ponds. These ponds would impound and store the runoff from the rainy season for use during the dry season, kind of like giant rain barrels, or cisterns. The dikes would either have control structures, like our monk, or just have a *tropplein* (overflow or spillway). Two inches of rainfall, not an unusual amount for a typical afternoon storm, falling on one acre of land would be 55,000 gallons of water. During the rainy season, a dam could impound about two million gallons of water from a one-acre watershed. Having a more consistent, reliable water supply would help to stabilize the food supply by allowing farmers to grow crops below the dams that would be irrigated by water from the reservoirs. I envisioned these hillside ponds dotting the savanna, providing year-round, life-giving water to the region. If my director had told me I would have been given all I needed to build as many hillside ponds as possible in a year, I would likely have stayed on to do it. Since I did not, the only reason I mention it now is in the hope that some future leader of the CAR, maybe some strong and determined village woman, will read this and say, *Let's do it!*

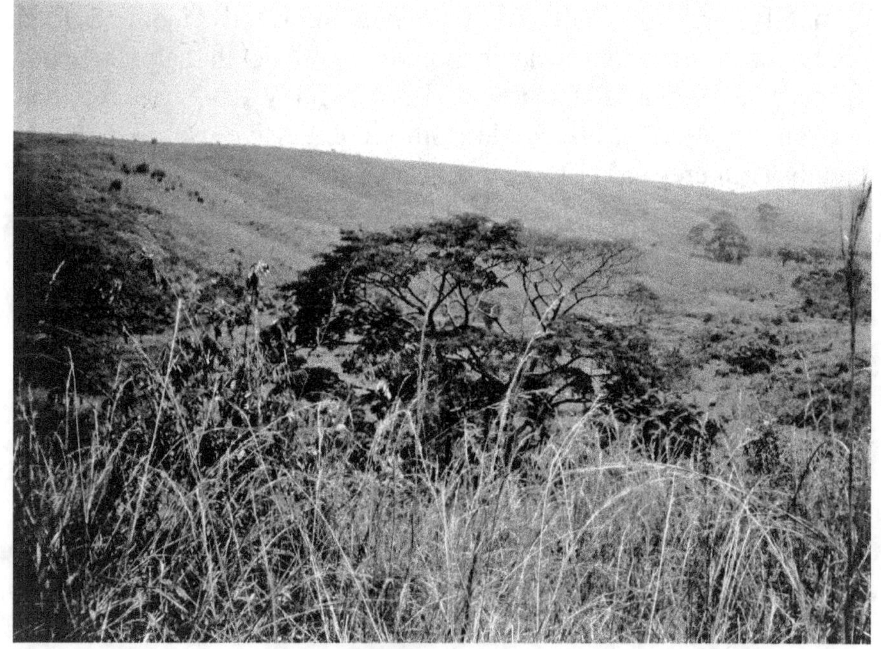

The spectacular Basse Kotto

When our family moved from Southwestern Florida, where I had worked as an environmental specialist in surface water management, to central New York, we were a family of three and Conor was a toddler. Peg worked full time (roughly nine days a week) as a nurse while Conor and I hung out and watched the two episodes of *Barney* that we had on VHS, interspersed with *Winnie the Pooh* and *The Little Mermaid*. After three years of this, however, I began to get restless. I started reading (these were, of course, pre-internet days) all I could get my hands on about recirculating, intensive tank culture of tilapia. Whether it was a blessing or a curse, I was only about two hours away from Cornell University, which was, at the time, pioneering many of the tank culture techniques for tilapia.

So, with Conor settled in with two hours of Winnie the Pooh and tethered to me electronically with a baby monitor, I added an insulated, passive-solar heated room to the back of our garage (with propane backup). I then designed and built a tank system capable of producing 2,000 pounds of tilapia every six months. I sold the tilapia at the Farmers Market in Cooperstown. The project, although it cost us about $10,000, accomplished its goal of giving me something to do. Without going into great detail about its construction and operation, I must say that it worked surprisingly well—at least for the first year and a half.

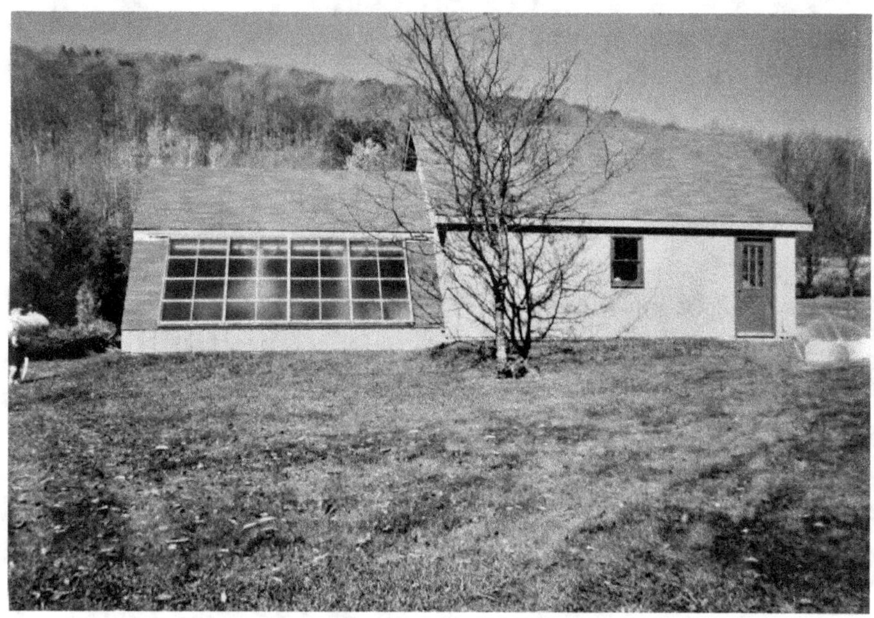

Insulated greenhouse behind our garage-1995

One side benefit of the system was the ability to add fish waste to our gardens. We had a plot of border-less raised beds adjacent to the building and a hose leading from the cone-shaped settling tank to the garden. The feces would settle out in the tank and fill the cone-shaped bottom. A valve was then opened every day to drain off the fluidized feces. In the summer, we were able to run this sludge directly onto the gardens, kind of like primitive aquaponics. The result was lettuce the likes of which I had never seen before, as well as massive leeks and bunching onions. I became well known at the farmers market for my leeks, and one customer I will never forget, a movie-star-looking blonde gal from Germany, came every week, just for my leeks. Peg did not necessarily share my enthusiasm for her patronage, nor did she think I was funny when I referred to myself as *The Scallion Stallion.*

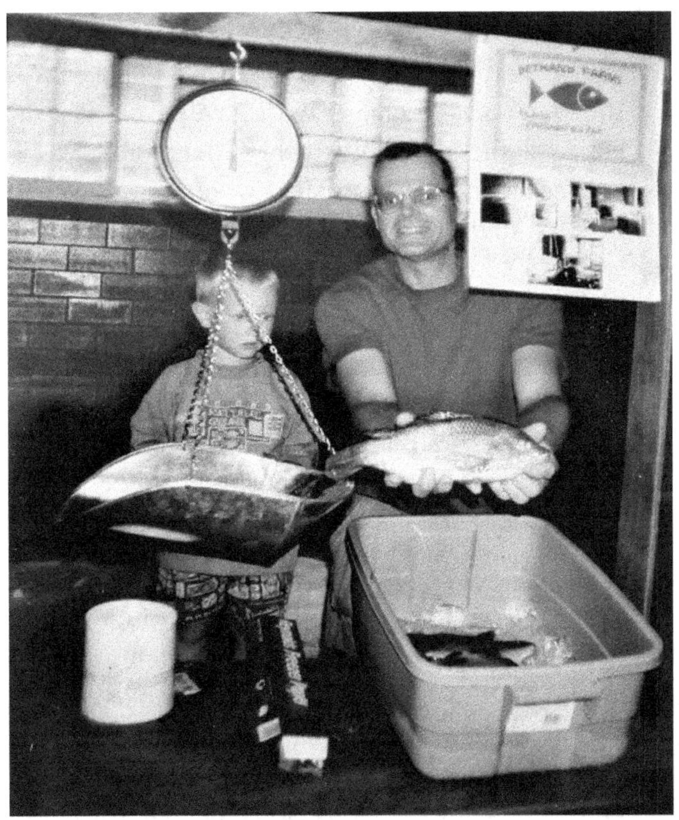

Me and Conor vending tilapia at the Farmers Market in Cooperstown, NY 1995

Being a shoestring-budgeted operation, we did not have a dedicated well for the aquaculture system; we simply ran a water line to it from the house. I also did not have the necessary funds for an automatic backup generator, should we lose power. It was always a nerve-wracking experience leaving the farm for a few hours. Conor and I once came home from a shopping trip to find that we had lost power and thousands of pairs of fish lips were piping for air on the surface. We were minutes away from a massive fish kill, so I ran our small portable generator to operate the blower until power was restored.

The crushing blow came during our second summer of operation when we had a drought that was severe enough to turn our lawn brown and crunchy, and finally affect our deep well. Our water turned yellow and gritty, and we were perilously close to losing our well. I was therefore only able to exchange less than five percent of the water in the tanks, and so we also had to cut way back on feed to avoid dangerously high ammonia levels. Then there was a severe thunderstorm that knocked out power for three days. I spent three nights sleeping on a cot in the garage, waking every two hours to add gas to the generator that was loud enough to be heard three miles away.

Fish farming was beginning to lose some of its glamour, and we had to make the decision to either invest in a dedicated deeper well for the fish farm and install an automatic backup generator or get out of the fish farming business. With great sadness, I sold the tanks and equipment for pennies on the dollar and chalked it up as an expensive life lesson.

Now I had a vacant insulated greenhouse and a lot of time on my hands, a potentially dangerous combination. I felt a great need to put this space to good use, but an even greater need to not spend any money doing it. Peg, interestingly, shared both the desire to find something for me to do, and to not spend any money doing it. The solution soon became obvious. I would build a hydroponics system. The aquaculture supply catalog, which had been my constant companion for a few years now, had a turnkey hydroponic system available for only $10,000. Turnkey obviously was not going to cut it, so I applied some appropriate-technology-type thought to it and whittled the cost down to $85. Since this would occupy a good chunk of my time, Peggy enthusiastically agreed that I should spend the whole $85 on plastic gutters, a small submersible pump, perlite, foam board, plastic tubs, tubing, fittings, and some plastic cups.

My homemade system of gutters, capped with foam board and drilled with holes every six inches for net pots, had a 400-plant capacity. Net pots are the perforated containers that hold the plant. They are filled with an inert media, in my case perlite (a white, lightweight volcanic mineral), and the seed germinates right in the pot. The roots then grow through the openings to reach the nutrient solution in the gutters. Back then, however, net pots were an expensive specialty item, and were outside of my budget. I had to make my own pots by cutting the bottoms from small plastic cups, securing squares of netting from the fabric shop to them using rubber bands, and filling them with perlite. Fabricating 400 of these single-use net pots proved to be a bit tedious. I had lots of time on my hands, but that does not mean that I enjoy tedious, repetitious work.

When I informed Peg that I may have gone a bit overboard by trying to grow 400 lettuce plants, she was not overly surprised. Nor was she shocked to hear that my lettuce was not as marketable or as valuable as I had anticipated. There was an upscale restaurant nearby, however, that specialized in freshly made pesto, so I made the shrewd business decision to switch to growing basil, which grew well in my system. It only paid enough, though, to purchase more Winnie the Pooh tapes.

I still enjoy dabbling in hydroponics, but I no longer rely on a pump submerged in a container below the gutters to deliver water back up to a reservoir above the gutters. We now use a non-circulating method that relies on an air space in the container between the water surface and the bottom of the net pot to supply oxygen to the roots. It is popularly known as the Kratky Method, named for the developer Dr. Bernard Kratky at the University of Hawaii. Anyone interested in this simple, productive way to grow greens needs only to search for the wealth of information about it on the internet.

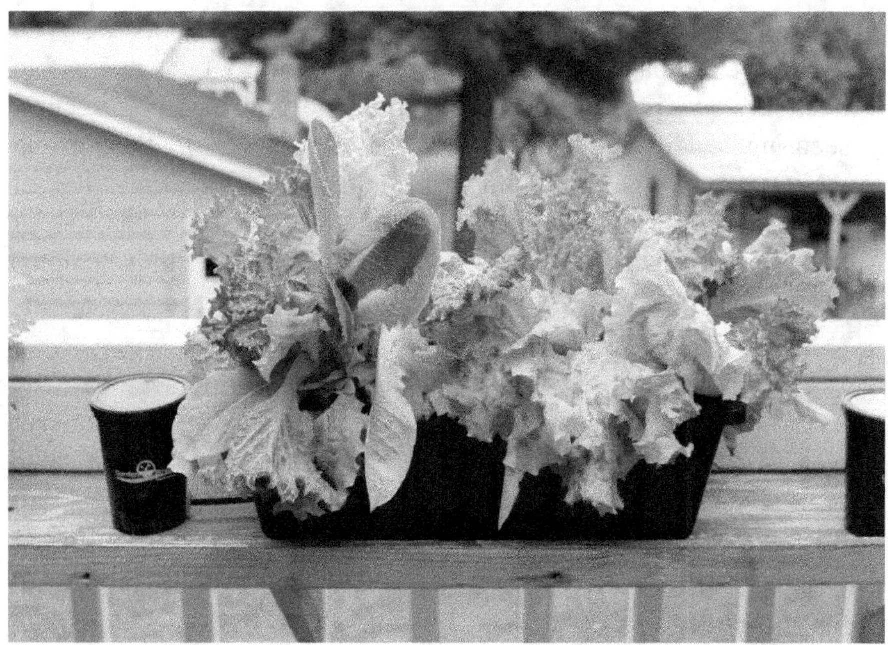

Hydroponics unplugged-our non-circulating system

We have now developed an automated, noncirculating hydroponic planter for growing greens both indoors and outdoors, using our Garden Stream™ system. Growing hydroponically outdoors, unless under cover, has its challenges. Most lids collect rainwater, which dilutes the nutrient solution. Our covers greatly reduce the infiltration of rainwater, and if a downpour does get into the planter, there are overflow holes to prevent flooding. Once again, we are happy to share our methods and hear about ideas for improving our methods.

Organic gardeners tend to look down on hydroponics as an artificial method that results in an incomplete, unbalanced, and less-nutritious plant. This may be true, and I agree that the best way to grow plants is in a living soil. But there are worse things that we could be eating than absolutely-fresh, pesticide-free produce.

Hydroponics can also be a big user of energy. To be commercially viable, the large growers must use artificial lighting and heat to mimic ideal growing conditions in their greenhouses, regardless of the conditions outside. To even consider hydroponics in northern Minnesota in the deep winter is, in my opinion, silly. But the appeal of such a system is its potential to grow 200 tons of produce per acre, as opposed to one ton per acre outside in the ground.

THE CLIMATE TAMER

A greenhouse operation that requires supplemental heat is not something that we are interested in considering as part of our operation. In the fall of 2016, I used two sliding glass door panels that I got for free from a friend to build a fifty-dollar solar heater that hangs on the south side of our house. The wooden box with foam board insulation and aluminum window screen stretched a couple of inches inside of the glass to trap the heat works amazingly well. A six-inch duct fan, activated by a thermal switch inside the heater, draws air from the basement and blows it into our upstairs kitchen. During its passage through the heater, the air warms from 60 degrees to over 150 degrees all for free. Back-draft preventers on each end (mostly) prevent cold air from infiltrating the house when the sun is not shining.

The trouble with anything that relies on solar energy in northern Minnesota is that there are many days or even weeks when the sun is not shining. It was not until we began operating the solar heater that we paid so much attention to the number of overcast winter days. From mid-November through December, we can go for weeks at a time without any heat coming from the solar heater. Once the arctic highs of January arrive, the solar heater earns its keep by pumping out air that is sometimes almost 200 degrees warmer than the outside temperature, even when it is -30 degrees outside. During those stretches of overcast days in the dead of winter, greenhouses (even the currently trendy deep-winter greenhouses) should, I believe, take a rest just as we do.

I do see the value of a *shallow winter* greenhouse, however, and hope to build one along the south side of our garage once I can locate enough free sliding door panels. I would insulate the floor using foamboard and cover it with gravel to provide some thermal mass. I would insulate the sloping shed roof and would provide very little if any supplemental heat. There would be a door on each end, which would mostly remain open in the summer months. The nearly vertical thermal panes would capture the low winter sunlight but would be mostly ignored by the high summer sun. I see this as an ideal place to start lettuce, microgreens, and herbs in late February, some heat-loving crops in the summer, and cold-tolerant greens once again in the fall. But from November through January, it would just be a storage room.

We would not be without our inexpensive, unheated hoop houses, however. For us zone 3 gardeners, the "days to maturity" numbers on the seed packets are serious business. Because frosts are common through May, and August is unreliable as well, a hoop house becomes a haven for aspiring seedlings and tender plants. We start our seeds in flats that sit atop soil-warming cables inside of cold frames that are, themselves, inside of the hoop house. The cold frame lids are also fitted with automatic vent openers, which perfectly complement the warming cables. When the soil temperature in the box drops below about seventy-two degrees, the cables turn on. When the sun warms the inside of the box past seventy-two degrees, the cables turn off and the lid begins to open to prevent overheating. All we need to do is sprinkle the tender seedlings with water to keep them moist. Tomato, pepper, and eggplant seedlings remain cozily growing, even during a March blizzard. We presently have two hoop houses in operation. They are 12' x 24' with 8' of headroom, and they each cost about $350 to construct.

Once it is safe to do so, the plants intended to grow outside in our raised beds are planted. The heat-loving plants, such as tomatoes, peppers, eggplant, basil, and some melons, will spend their entire lives inside of the hoop houses. Three of our fifty-gallon composters also reside inside the hoop houses. We generally have no need for fertilizers or weed or pest control in this environment. The doors on each end remain propped open during the day throughout the summer unless the forecast calls for a cold snap.

We generally enjoy fresh produce from the hoop houses well into October. In fact, we are usually sick of tomatoes and peppers well before they succumb to frost.

The mental health benefits from owning a hoop house should also not be overlooked. By mid- March, winter is losing some of its charm for most of us, and it generally does not help to see the beach photos of our tanned, smiling friends visiting Florida or Mexico. A hoop house can provide a mini vacation that is much cheaper and more convenient than a trip to Florida, and will give us a tan that rivals the $2,000 ones that our friends are sporting. A lounge chair, a beverage appropriate for the time of day, and a good book is all that is required to bask in eighty-plus degree temperatures as we reintroduce our pasty skin to the first rays of sunlight in five months. One word of caution, however, should you be one to want to maximize the amount of skin being exposed to the sunlight: the translucent greenhouse film covering the hoop house is more revealing than one might think—especially on a bright, sunny day. It sure feels good, though, to be basking in Florida-caliber weather when it is twenty degrees outside.

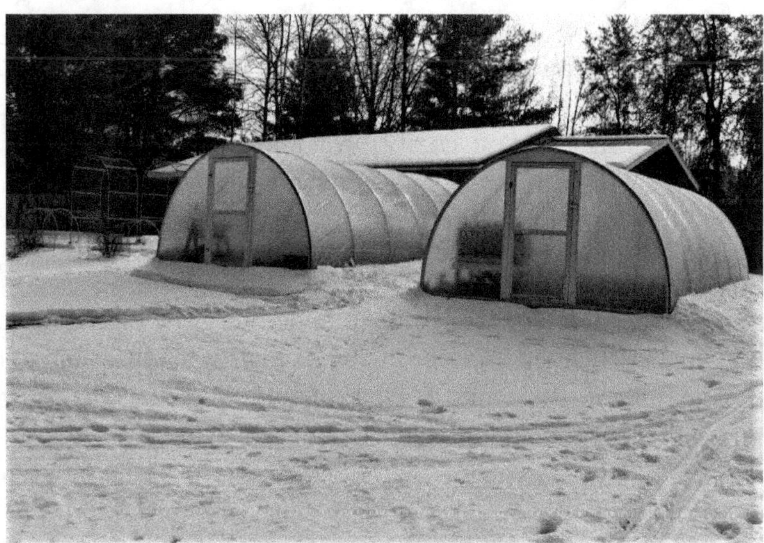

The hoop houses taking a break in the winter

THE GARDENSTREAM

I am giving an overview of what we do not only to boast, but also to point out that growing some of your own food can be both fun and rewarding. The hoop houses, composters, raised beds, chicken cages, and self-watering planters are all products that we make and use ourselves. Since not everyone has an interest in all, or any, of these designs, I have chosen not to include the detailed construction plans in this book. If I have inspired anyone to want to learn more, please contact us, and we will gladly share our designs. One product though, stands out as being at the heart of our gardening operation. It is one that allows anyone with a level surface in the sun to enjoy gardening. Remember way back, when I referred to a garden as a wellness center? Well, we sincerely believe that, and our mission is to make gardening as accessible to as many as possible by making it as simple as possible.

We came up through the ranks of home gardening much the same as most gardeners. At one point, we had over 2,400 square feet of garden beds that were tilled using a rear-tined rototiller. We used a walk-behind seeder to plant row after row of crops, followed by cultivating, weeding, watering, weeding, thinning, and weeding. At the end of it all, there was the harvest of much more produce than we could possibly consume or process. It did not stop us from trying, however. Thirty quarts of watery salsa may seem ridiculous to us now, but back then it gave us bragging rights. Our good friends down the road were putting up thirty-five quarts of watery salsa a year, so the only thing to do was to keep expanding our operation. Gardening was becoming a competitive sport.

Perhaps it was through divine intervention, but suddenly some glossy brochures for a self-watering planter began showing up in our mailbox. These plastic boxes had a four-gallon water reservoir covered with a perforated plastic false bottom. The box was filled with a non-mineral-based potting mix that rested above the water reservoir, except for two places where it could wick the water up to moisten the soil. No watering, no weeding, no pests, no tilling. The claims seemed too good to be true, so I bought a hundred of them. At $35 apiece (wholesale plus shipping), this was beginning to feel alarmingly like a tilapia operation. But I assured Peg that I had a sound business plan: I would buy $400 worth of composted pine bark, bales of peat, and sacks of perlite and fertilizer to make my own potting mix. I would then start tomato and pepper plants from seed and sell the planters already filled and planted with big, healthy plants. It would be a turnkey operation.

It took two years, but I finally sold eighty percent of the planters. That left us with twenty of them to use ourselves. During this first (and only) season of planting all twenty of them, we had containers lining every speck of our outdoor living space. It really was spectacular to look at. At first, these containers proved to be as productive as advertised. What the glossy brochures failed to mention, however, was that two mature tomato plants will consume more than four gallons of water in a day. We would come home from a relaxing afternoon on the lake only to find our massive tomato plants lying flat on the ground. I would then drag out the garden hose and, like filling gas tanks, top off all the reservoirs through the fill tubes. The plants would have mostly recovered by morning, but they never forgave us for our neglect. Besides our drought/deluge watering routine, we were immersing the warm, drying roots in fifty-degree well water. This was getting old too. This was feeling too much like the days of not being able to leave home for fear of losing thousands of fish. I knew that a float valve connected to a reliable water supply was in my future. Again, in the name of brevity—and sanity—I will omit the details of the four-year quest for the perfect device to automate our self-watering planters. The Garden Stream™ is what emerged, and that is what is important. It is a simple box containing an adjustable mini float valve connected to a water supply and a daisy-chain of downstream containers.

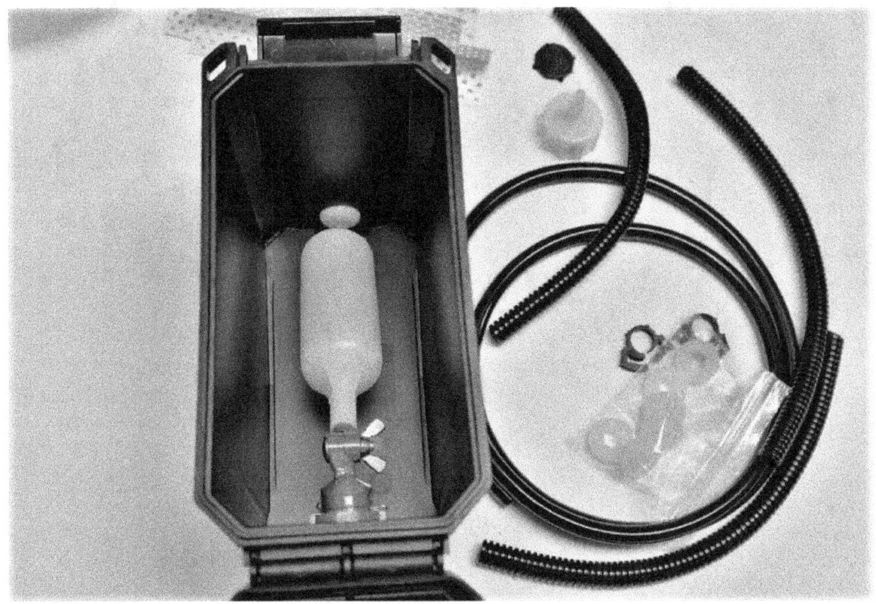

An adjustable mini float valve housed in a lidded box, connected to a water supply, will water our planters all season

All that is required is a level surface (since the water level must be the same throughout the system) and sunlight. With it, an urban grower can convert a deck, patio, sidewalk, driveway, or even a flat rooftop, to a garden, using about twenty percent of the water of a conventional garden. As important as gardening is for our bodies and our souls, being held captive by one is not much fun.

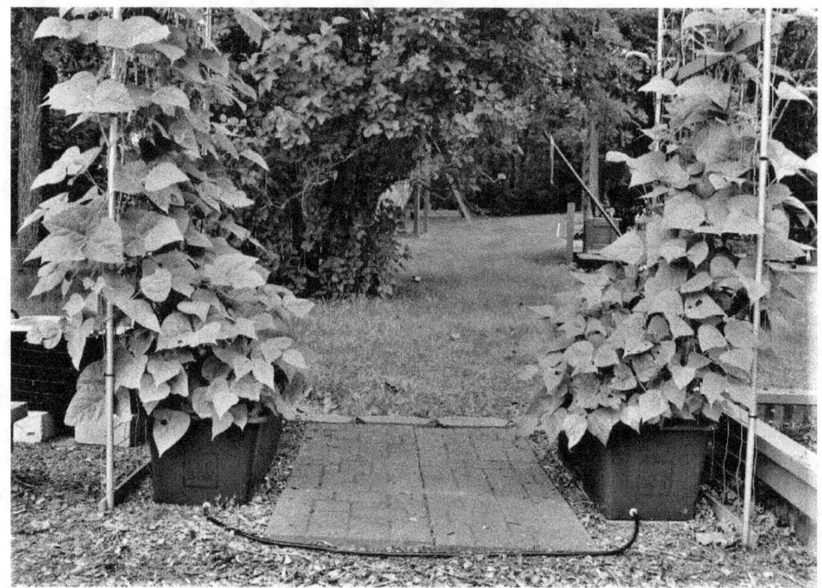

Bottom watering planters that self-water for weeks at a time

PASTURED POULTRY

We seldom buy meat from a store, although I admit to being partial to a good ham that I then sometimes double smoke to double the flavor. Locally sourced, naturally raised pork is ideal. Curing hams, unfortunately, is not done regionally like it once was. At one time, I did some custom curing of locally raised hams for customers, but that was back in the days when we had a $7,000 commercial smoker and a licensed sausage kitchen. Anyway, aside from pastured ham, we don't buy much meat. We do keep a steady supply of venison, fish, locally raised beef, and our own chickens in our freezer, however.

After reading Joel Salatin's book, *Pastured Poultry Profits*, in the 1990s, I was captivated by the idea of raising chickens in mobile cages. Even if you have no interest in raising chickens yourself, this book is worth reading just to make you aware of the backstory of the chicken that makes its way into our supermarkets and restaurants. Mr. Salatin does a very good job of opening our hearts and minds to the dark side of an industry that treats living creatures as a commodity that has the inconvenient habit of being alive. Once again, I will spare the details, since I am close to reaching my rant quota. Others are much more informed than I am on the topic, but I will just say that reading about it was enough to make me *not* want to support the confinement industry by purchasing their products.

The superstar of meat birds is the Cornish Cross hybrid. The breed was developed in concert with the confinement production of poultry, which got rolling in the 1940s. As confinement production has pushed the limits, so has the refinement of the birds raised in these limit-pushing facilities. This hybrid has since been bred for unnaturally rapid growth, amazingly efficient conversion rates, massive breasts, and sparse feathering, to reach an average dressed weight of five pounds in six to seven weeks. These birds have more-or-less had *being a chicken* bred out of them, leaving them prone to all sorts of ailments and conditions that are dealt with using antibiotics, hormones, and other medications in intensive confinement operations.

The Cornish Cross breed has become strictly a commodity: a feathered protein factory. I suspect that the dream of the factory poultry operators would be to breed a featherless creature that could remain strapped on its back to a conveyor belt, with a feeding tube and catheter installed, where it would remain from the day it hatched until the day it was conveyed to the processing facility. The growers could even route the conveyor belt over some nice, green grass so their marketers could label their products as *pastured poultry.*

The chicken I grew up eating was more like the chicken I had in the CAR than like what is available in the supermarkets today. My grandparents had hundreds of laying hens and were wholesalers of eggs. Those hens were not confined in cages but were allowed the run of a former cattle barn that had wooden nest boxes lining its walls. In the summer, the hens could venture outdoors in a fenced area. I have mostly fond memories of helping Grandpa collect eggs in the morning. I say *mostly* because, although it felt good to reach under the warm body of a brooding hen to extract the warm eggs from beneath her feathered body, the occasional peck I received from a noncompliant hen made me a bit apprehensive. Once we had our baskets full, the eggs would be carried back to the big farm kitchen, where they would be hand-washed, allowed to dry in large mesh baskets, and then brought down into the cellar, where they would be misted with mineral oil and crated for shipment to the co-op.

The chickens I grew up eating were the underperforming hens or the odd surly rooster. Grandma would grab the leg snare that hung inside the door, deftly hook the victim by its leg and, with no hesitation, take it outside, chop off its head, pluck, eviscerate, and rinse the carcass at the well house for the evening meal. Now that was fresh poultry. That chicken may not have been super tender, but it was packed with flavor. The muscles were well developed with a striated texture, and the bones were hard, white, and translucent. Grandma's oven-fried chicken baked long enough to make even a tough old rooster reasonably tender and flavorful.

This is what I expected our own Cornish Cross chickens to taste like when we processed our first batch. It was a puzzling disappointment, though, to bite into soft, rather mushy meat that was lacking that real-chicken flavor; and the bones, too, were mushy, and dark- colored. This was the trade-off we were going to have to contend with if we did not want to spend our entire summer tending slower-growing chickens. A Cornish Cross, at seven weeks, is not yet a mature bird. What we are eating are giant chicks that have not yet lived long enough for their muscles to mature and develop full flavor and texture.

As a trial, one season we raised Red Rangers, a slower-growing hybrid. These birds were excellent foragers and fun birds to work with. In flavor and texture, they were similar to Grandma's chicken, and the bones were white, hard, and translucent. But they took a month longer, were expensive to buy and feed and, in the end, we had birds that dressed out at three to four pounds.

We usually raise the Cornish Cross breed now and rationalize that we are, at least, eating an all- natural chicken that was well treated, and had lived a contented life up until that last day. This past season, we experimented, and raised fourteen Cornish Cross and eleven Red Rangers. I had an opportunity to buy eleven two-week-old Red Ranger chicks and could not pass it up. The next day I bought fourteen-day-old Cornish Cross chicks. One of them died within hours, and three more of them died during the grow-out period. One of them actually keeled-over from an apparent heart attack while I was watching it. It is disheartening to see mostly grown birds become crippled and die. So, the one-dollar-per-bird cost savings for the Cornish Cross gets wiped out when they die like that. We did not lose a single Red Ranger. Only four of them were hens, which we kept as layers. Don't let anyone tell you that Rangers are poor layers. Ours have been superb layers, and some of the most pleasant chickens to have around. The dress-out weight of the Red Rangers was a pound or so less, even though they were two weeks older. If the quantity of meat is the goal, go with the Cornish. If high-quality meat is the goal, stick with the Rangers.

Our mobile pen design is 10' x 6', with an arched center height of 3'. About two-thirds of the mesh top is covered with a tarp to provide shade and refuge from the rain. The pens are lightweight, inexpensive to construct, and quite durable. They are also so easy to move that a child can do it. The capacity is about twenty-five birds.

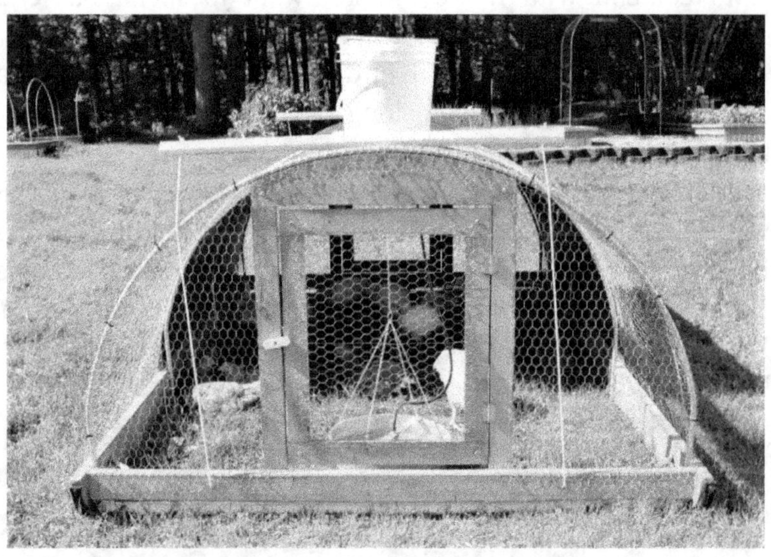

Our 6'x10' mobile cage with automatic waterer

Now, some may say that we are cruel to confine twenty-five chickens in a sixty-square-foot space. But we must remember that the Cornish Cross has such ponderous breasts that simply walking can be a struggle for them. During their lives in overcrowded indoor confinement, they just slide across a feces-encrusted floor to get to the feed and water, breathing air that is thick with fecal dust. Our chickens get fresh grass underfoot every day, two to three times per day as they mature. They always have a supply of clean water and, like manna from heaven, feed that gets sprinkled through the cage top every day. They can also forage for insects and fresh grass, should they choose to do so. *Being a chicken* may have been bred out of them, but their latent survival instinct is revived a bit once these birds are freed from the horrors of the confinement barns. They walk taller and even strut and test their wings as they revel in fresh air, fresh water, fresh grass, insects, and wholesome food. It is fun to watch the transformation, and we are rewarded with meat that is as good as the breed can offer us.

We may not save money by raising our own chickens but knowing how they were raised makes it worth the effort. For those who want chicken as part of their diet but have no desire to raise and process them themselves, there is the option of purchasing chickens from a grower who raises them in a conscientious manner. For those who do have an interest in raising their own chickens, feel free to contact us and we will gladly share our plans and experiences.

The float valve we use to automate our self-watering planters also can be used to make an automatic hanging waterer that travels with the cage and is fed by water from a bucket strapped to the cage top. An added benefit of pastured poultry is that the former cage site soon becomes lush lawn. The cage may also be placed over a garden plot and the remains can be worked into the soil. We rake the leavings from a former cage site into our composters, which gets things heating up in no time and contributes to rich compost.

PADDLE YOUR OWN CANOE

To *paddle your own canoe* refers to charting your own course, taking charge of your own life, and pursuing your dreams... Or it might just mean building your own canoe and paddling it. Our son Conor and I built two stitch-and-tape solo canoes back when he was a young teen. These were lightweight (about thirty-pound) canoes built from thin, marine-grade tropical hardwood plywood called *okoume*. Due to the size constraints imposed by two sheets of plywood, however, they had an unsettlingly narrow beam and so little freeboard that we became a bit too intimate with the water surface. We had built these canoes intending to take them into the Boundary Waters Canoe Area Wilderness (BWCAW) in northeastern Minnesota. After a few sea trials, however, we realized that they didn't have the capacity for both ourselves and our gear. This prompted a quest to design and build my own dream canoe, one I named *Ripple*. I wrote a book on its construction, should anyone be interested in building a fourteen-foot wood and fiberglass canoe in about forty hours for about $300. The book is titled: *Making a Ripple-the 2x4 Canoe* (end of plug).

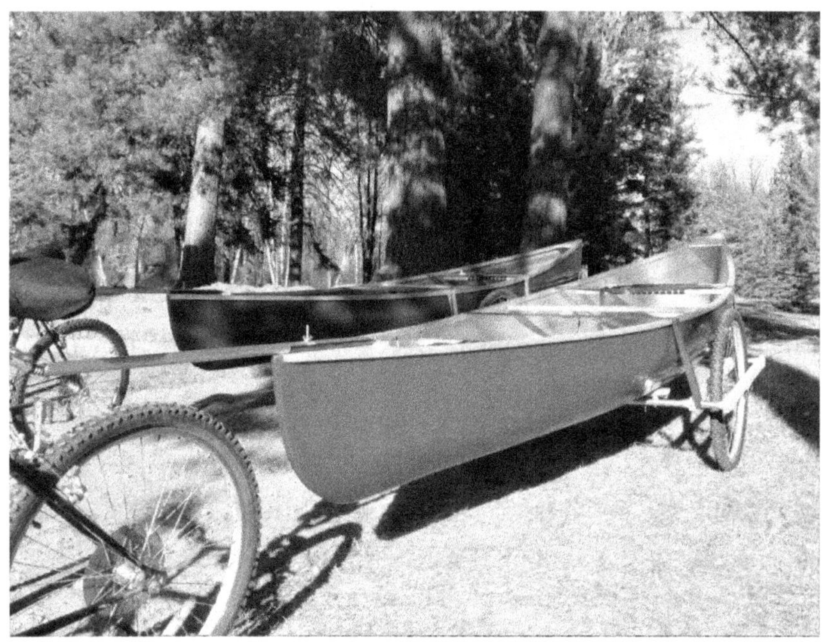

Two of my Ripples on bike trailers

What prompted our foray into the world of canoe building was our first trip into the BWCAW when Conor was fifteen years old. This was a trip arranged through our church, and it was intended to be a youth/parent trip. When we arrived at the base camp, however, Conor and I were surprised to learn that, out of the entire state, Conor was the only youth and I was the only parent who had signed up for this trip. Our guides were two young college gals who made a quick assessment of youth, stamina, vitality, and sinewy brawn. Then they glanced at Conor and made a similar assessment. This was the chance they had been waiting for. Up until now, they had to plan leisurely routes to accommodate a variety of skill levels. But not now. They were taking us on the route they had been hoping to take all summer but, having been constrained by mere mortals, had been unable to.

Our first lesson was to never pack all the items on the list that we had so meticulously studied at home. I should have learned this lesson from my initial packing for the CAR, but that experience had been long forgotten. We each had two pairs of blue jeans, spare sneakers, sweatshirts, socks, spare underwear, pajamas, Conor's hard-covered bible, and rain gear (and this was not summer rain gear, but our heavy-duty October duck-hunting rain gear). All this gear had to fit into one pack, which weighed in at more than eighty pounds. It was made from heavy, blue/gray synthetic canvas, and Conor dubbed it *Big Blue*. It turns out that we wore, every day and night, our swim trunks, water shoes, and a T-shirt. None of the other items, including Conor's bible, ever surfaced from the depths of Big Blue. We later made a mental note that our next trip would include a pair of lightweight nylon pants with removable leggings, water shoes, a T-shirt, sweatshirt, swim trunks, and a toothbrush with most of the handle sawed off.

Our canoe was made of Kevlar, was eighteen feet long, and weighed thirty-five pounds—less than half the weight of Big Blue. Our food was carried in a bear-resistant plastic barrel fitted with straps, so it could be carried on our backs. Conor quickly learned that the food barrel, unlike Big Blue, became noticeably lighter after each stop, so he volunteered to carry it. Big Blue actually got heavier, since loading a wet tent and wet sleeping bags into it each morning added several pounds to the pack.

About noon, we would begin to seek a suitable lunch spot, which usually was a large, gently sloping rock that provided easy access, a nice lounging surface, and a good swim platform. The BWCAW is unique because it consists of more water than dry land. There is enough dry land, however, to interfere with paddling. We were therefore interrupted several times a day by portages across these landmasses. For some reason, the US Forest Service, which manages the BWCAW, feels compelled to maintain ties to a bygone era by listing the lengths of these portages in *rods*. It did not matter that we arrived at the base camp in a modern vehicle and we were paddling a $2,400 canoe made from the same material used in bulletproof vests. When it came to the length of a portage, we were traveling back to the year 1725. It turns out that a rod is the approximate length of a 1725 model birch bark canoe, which was 16.5 feet. I wished many times that we had swapped out the pajamas for a pocket calculator. Converting rods to feet became a major pastime of mine as we paddled from portage to portage. Let's see, a 120-rod portage would be 120 x 16.5 =1980 feet, divided by 5280 feet = 0.375 miles. One-third of a mile doesn't sound like a long distance unless it is along a slippery, rock-strewn, narrow footpath while sporting Big Blue and carrying a 1.09-rod-long canoe.

The highlight of the day was our arrival at the campsite for the night and a well-deserved rest. First, we unpacked the wet tents and sleeping bags and hung them out to dry so they could re-hydrate overnight. Then we refilled our water bottles by wading into the lake to pump cool, clear lake water through the filters into water bottles (if only we had known about these pumps in the CAR, but more on that later). We then would go for a swim, and Conor and I would fish while the gals reposed and read books.

Our first dinner was to be a memorable one, especially for Conor. After paddling a good fifteen miles and making several long portages, a fifteen-year-old boy is ready for a good 6,000-calorie supper. Our petite guides, however, were woefully out of touch with the caloric needs of a growing boy as they busily prepared our tiny meal on a tiny stove in a tiny pot. The dinner was to be one of the *Helper* dinners that consist of a tiny pouch of elbow macaroni and a tinier foil pouch of powdered flavoring and thickener. This was the tuna version, so a single pouch of tuna (cans are not allowed into the BWCAW) was added to the cooked noodles and the powder. When Conor was handed his one-third-cup portion I thought he was going to cry. He could easily have consumed four of these entire boxed dinners by himself. But there was dessert, right? As a special treat, we were presented with a no-bake cheesecake dessert that had been reconstituted from powder containing an impressive ingredient list. I realized how truly awful this concoction was when Conor took one bite and spat it out. Despite his hunger, his real-food upbringing would not allow this stuff to enter his body.

Up to this point, we thought that we had brought our fishing gear along for recreational fishing. After that first meal at the hands of our guides, we realized that our ability to catch fish meant the difference between having an adequate supper and a very expensive and substantial weight-loss program. Since we had not signed up for a weight-loss program, we fished every afternoon and dined on some of the freshest fish that could be had anywhere in the world. Amazingly, our guides had not considered freshly caught fish as a menu item. They thought nothing of purchasing tuna, a threatened, mercury-laden apex predator that had been caught months earlier, packaged in Thailand, and shipped thousands of miles to become part of a meal in one of the most remote wilderness areas left in America. Dining on freshly caught smallmouth bass, northern pike, and walleye from the pristine lakes had, somehow, not entered their minds. Such is our conditioning to rely on supermarket food.

Conor and I went on one more church sponsored BWCAW canoe trip. This trip, however, included several other youths from our congregation, and I was one of the adult chaperones. We were hopeful that the hundreds of dollars we were spending on this trip would, this time, include adequate meals. Conor and I were not taking chances, however, and brought along our fishing gear. Thankfully we did, because the food situation—inexplicably—was not much improved. Had we not brought our fishing gear and supplemented every meal with fresh fish, there may have been a mutiny. Even with the added protein, our teenaged crew was left woefully wandering from tiny pot to tiny pot with empty plates, searching for any remaining morsels. Why the outfitters chose to scrimp on something as important and rewarding as a fulfilling meal remains a mystery. With careful planning, and especially with packaged meals made from dehydrated produce from our garden, a meal in the wilderness can be an inexpensive, rewarding, and memorable feast.

When I told Peg that I was writing about our wilderness experiences in the BWCAW, she looked doubtful and she pointed out that two such trips did not make me expert enough to give advice to others. This critique hurt a bit until it dawned on me that

I had, in fact, been on a wilderness canoe trip that few in America—perhaps even the world—had ever experienced. This trip of a lifetime was Tom's brainchild. He, Stewart, Mac, and I, along with a Central African guide, were to paddle a pirogue (dugout canoe) down the Oubangui River, from Mobaye to Bangui. I was informed of this plan when I returned to the CAR from my medical leave. When I balked, saying I had only been back in Mobaye long enough to lose my *bien engraissé* status, and had too much work to do, he explained that they had been waiting for me to get back before taking this trip, and that (this was the clincher) it would be the kind of trip to *tell my grandchildren about*. It turns out they also needed me to arrange for both the pirogue and the guide, Joseph, a Sango fisherman who had grown up on the river.

So, in the spring of 1984, during the dry season, the five of us embarked on an adventure that would be retold many times to my own children, and soon to our new grandson, Emmett. (Thank you, Tom.) Our craft was a nearly thirty- foot-long canoe that had been made by removing most of the interior from a massive tropical hardwood log. The incredibly labor-intensive task of hewing and burning the wood from this log resulted in a watercraft that must have weighed in at well over 1,000 pounds. With a forty-inch beam, the canoe had enough stability for us to walk around in it once we had our sea legs. Having room for five crew members and all of our gear came at the expense of responsiveness, however. Fittingly, our paddles were also carved from dense, heavy hardwood. There were to be no portages on this trip.

The only time a trip such as this can be safely navigated is during the dry season, when the water level drops substantially from its bank-filling, rainy season torrent. During the dry season, there is a considerable amount of seasonal real estate, in the form of sandbars, providing us endless lunch stop and campsite options. There is also little current, except for in the narrows, which made for safer travels, but offered little assistance in propelling our massive craft 400 kilometers to Bangui.

Joseph carried along a large cooking pot and the necessary utensils for our meal preparation. Unlike our BWCAW guides, Joseph knew he could rely on fresh fish for the bulk of our meals. We also packed rice and manioc, peanut butter, hot pepper powder, onion, garlic, and palm oil. I was the only crew member who brought along fishing tackle, so we bought freshly netted fish from passing Sango fishermen. As was customary in the CAR, we would arrive at a suitable sandbar—preferably one on a bank with overhanging trees to provide some shade—for the main meal and a well-deserved rest. As Joseph went off in search of three rocks and some firewood, cleaned the fish, and got the meal cooking, the rest of us would go for a swim and refill our water jugs. I would then do some fishing. While I was back home, I had the foresight to pack one of my heavy muskie fishing rods and some muskie lures.

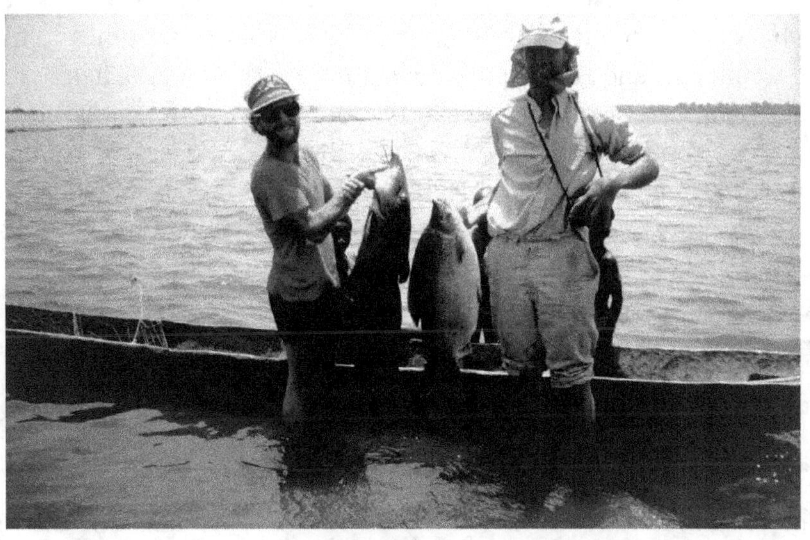

Stewart (left) and Mac, checking out possible dinner menu items

During one of these noon stops I waded out with my fishing gear and began throwing a large spinnerbait, while Joseph tended the fire and my other crew members lounged in the shade. Suddenly, I let out a whoop as something big hit my lure. Before I could react and loosen my drag, the fish had buried the thirty-six-pound braided Dacron line deep into the spool. I could not let any line out as the most powerful fish I had (or have) ever encountered pulled me into deeper water. As the line tightened like piano wire and I was about to be pulled onto my face in the water, the surface erupted as a one-hundred-pound tigerfish tail-danced on the water. As its massive, silvery side slapped back to the surface, the line snapped and I was left standing chest-deep in the water, looking back to shore where four slack-jawed men stood staring. By not first checking my drag, I had missed out on the chance of landing the fish of a lifetime and becoming a local legend. But it was too big to keep anyway. I then redeemed myself slightly by tying on another leader and lure and catching a much smaller, but still fierce-looking and quite-tasty, tigerfish. None of us were inclined to go for our customary noon swim at that beach.

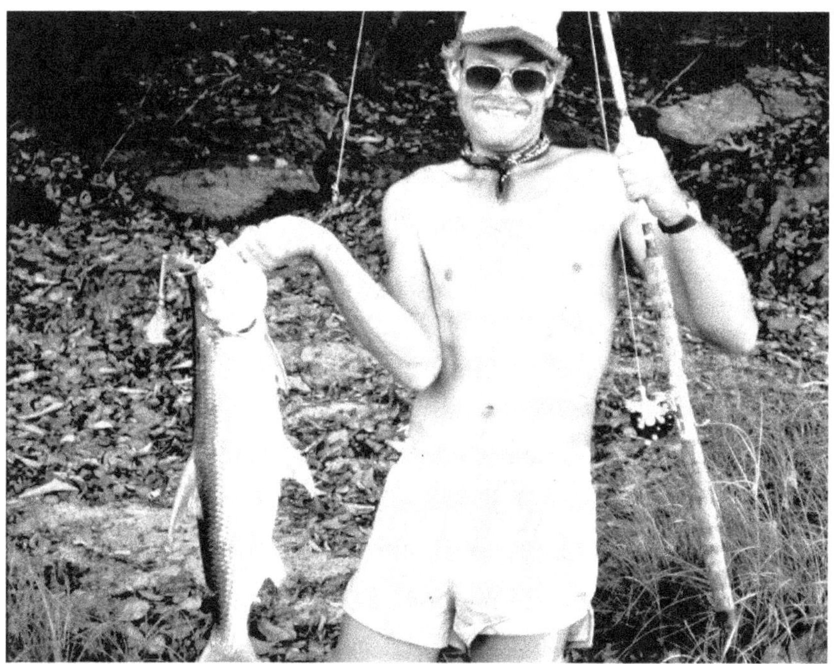

The little Tigerfish I caught to redeem myself after losing the monster

One food item that I recall vividly is dates. Tom had somehow acquired bags and bags of dried dates. We ate dates all day long, every day, until we were all sick of dates. In fact, those were the only dates we ended up having for quite some time. Now, thirty-six years later, I still shiver at the thought of eating dried dates.

It is amazing how much water five men paddling a thousand-pound canoe through still waters under the equatorial sun can consume in a day. We filled three or four five-gallon plastic jerry cans each day and dissolved iodine tablets in them to purify the water. It was Tom's job to bring both the dates and the iodine tablets, and, erring on the cautious side, he brought along two bottles of tablets. About mid-way through the trip, however, it was discovered that Tom's foray into the world of responsibility had not included looking inside of the bottles to verify that they did, in fact, contain iodine tablets. The second bottle was empty, which left us in a bit of a predicament: should we keelhaul him or make him walk the plank?

Being too fatigued to do any of that, we pulled onto a sandbar to consider how we were going to get our drinking water for the next four days without a means of sanitizing it. Stewart, being from California (along with Mac), had access to technology that Tom and I, being from Minnesota, had not heard of. Stewart had brought along, for example, a tube with some lotion called *sunscreen*, and applied it to his skin. Tom and I, being more resourceful, simply tied water-soaked bandanas to our south-facing upper arms to reduce the blistering. But Stewart had heard that digging a hole in the sand and allowing the water to slowly fill the hole resulted in sand-filtered water. So, we got busy, using our paddles to dig holes in the sand, and watched as water quickly gushed in to fill them. We scooped the turbid, gritty water into our jugs, and continued-on our journey. We had the good fortune the following day to find a spring along a steep bank of the river, with clear water flowing freely from it. We dumped our sandy water and filled every container we had with what was to be the last pure water of the trip.

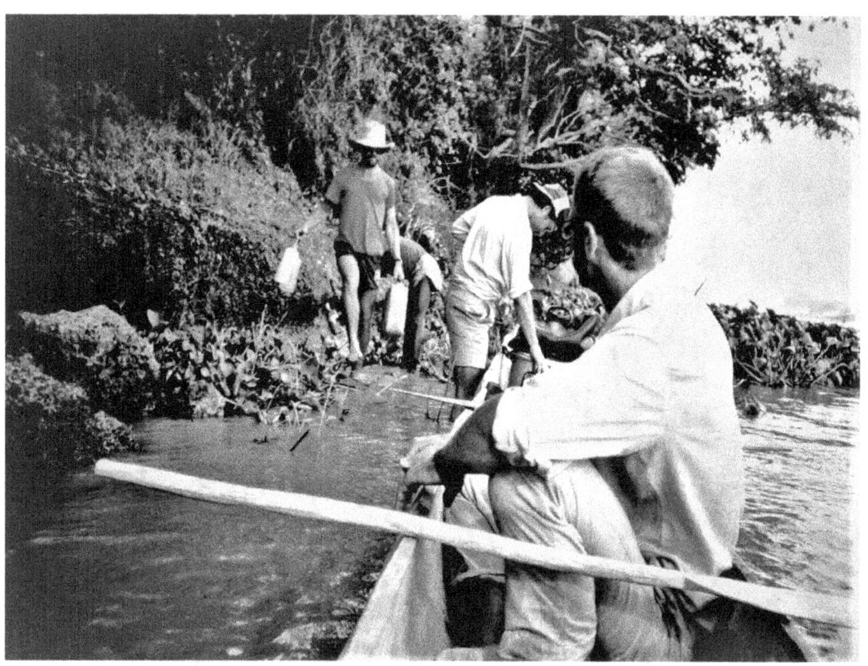

Filling every jug we had with fresh spring water for the last clean water of the trip

When the water level drops several feet from its rainy season levels, the Sango fishermen move their entire villages out onto the island sandbars. These seasonal island villages consisted of small, domed huts made from woven palm fronds, and they even moved their livestock—usually goats and chickens—out with them. We spent our nights on these same sandbars, sharing in the hospitality of the villagers. We slept on woven mats laid out on the sand, under mosquito netting suspended from the paddles stuck into the sand as corner posts.

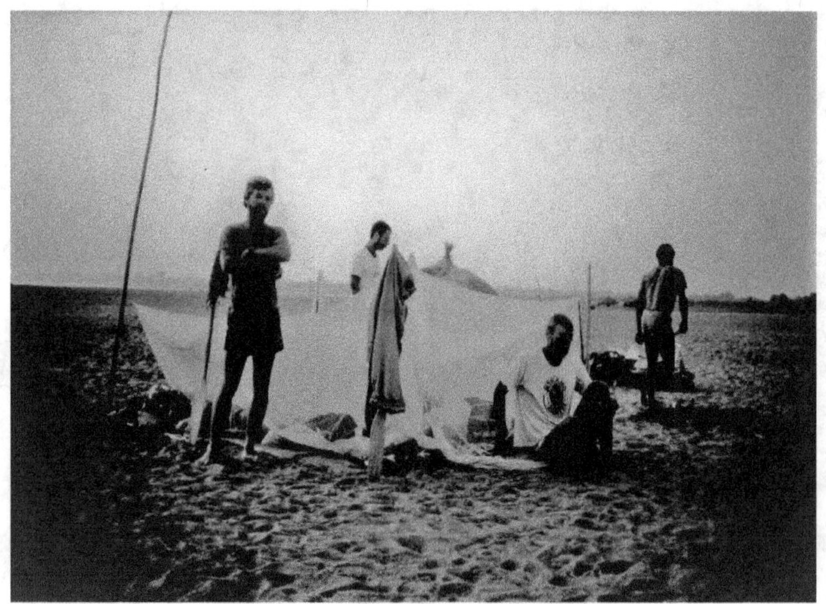

Setting up camp for the night on a sandbar

One memorable night stands out because of a rare dry-season thunderstorm. Although infrequent during the dry season, when they did occur, they were spectacular. This was one such storm, and it was a vulnerable feeling being the high point on a sandbar in the middle of a broad expanse of the river with lightning seemingly all around us. The Sango knew what to expect and invited us to seek refuge in their humble abodes. Although it was cramped quarters, and not likely much of a haven from lightning strikes, we gratefully welcomed the cozy escape from the torrential downpour outside.

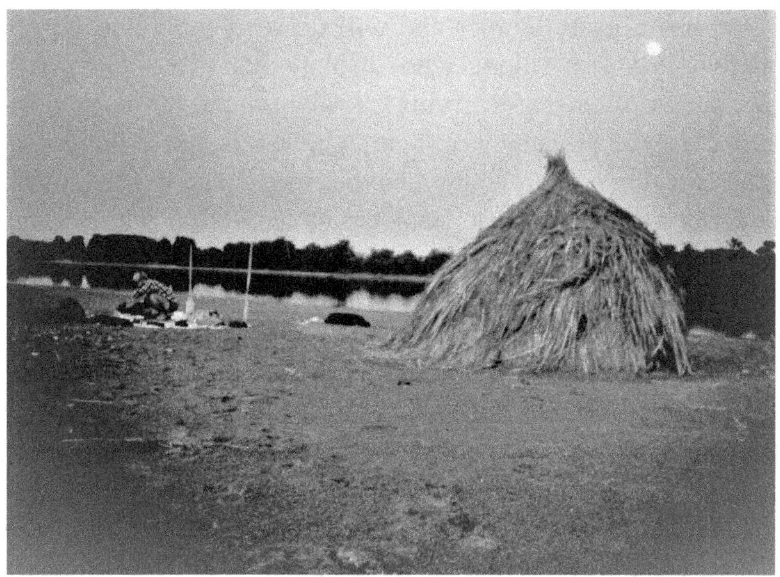

Typical Sango hut like the one that saved us from a wild storm

We were able to repay the kindness of the Sango by leaving the next village downstream with a tale that would no doubt be told around the evening fires for years to come. As sunset approached, we began searching for a sandbar where we could spend the night. Up ahead, in the middle of the river, was a long, narrow sandbar with a Sango village on its lower end. My knee was still not fully mended, and it stiffened up after a day of paddling, so I asked to be dropped off at the top of the sandbar to walk off the stiffness. I would then meet up with the crew at the lower end. Since darkness was fast approaching, I noted that the evening fires were already being tended in front of the huts, and families were gathering around them. Apparently, due to their preoccupation with this evening ritual, our approach had gone undetected by anyone in the village.

There are legends among the people of Africa of a white spirit, called *Mami Wata*, which has special meaning to the Sango fishermen. The word is of English origin, being derived from *Mommy Water*, and likely originated in West Africa. In the CAR, it refers to a white female with long, straight hair, who has the power to heal the sick and bring good tidings to her believers. But she also has a nasty temper and will drown people and do other vindictive things to those who disobey her. To make matters worse, she is often seen carrying a snake around her neck, just in case she is not already scary enough. I was not a long-haired woman carrying a snake, but when the first person to see me was a poor child who happened to look up to see a very white, skinny, bearded creature limping right toward him, it made sense for him to believe that he was about to be eaten. As he shrieked with pure terror, his cries were soon echoed by every child within sight of this apparition. (I think there may have also been a few adults joining in.) It was not until the canoe was spotted that it made sense who I was and where I came from. Once it was known that the canoe was headed for a landing at the lower end of the sandbar, the sheer terror was switched off and was replaced by intense curiosity, and the entire village ran to greet the crew.

As the canoe made landfall, with the bow digging into the sandbar, the villagers were already assembled, seated on the sloping sand as if in a stadium. First Tom, Stewart, and then Joseph wearily made their way to the bow and crawled over it carrying their gear. This left Mac alone near the stern. At about 6'6" in height, Mac was a tall man, even by American standards. Since Central Africans are not tall people, Mac towered over everyone. He also had a head of white-blond hair and looked to me like someone from California was supposed to look. But Mac was weary from a full day of paddling and was perhaps a bit grumpy. So, when he stood up, he did not even acknowledge the gasps of amazement and excited chatter due to his towering build. Mac just slung his pack over his shoulder, stepped over the gunwale into the water...*and completely disappeared from view*. All that remained of all 6'6" of Mac was his cap floating on the surface. While the near-shore waters were fairly shallow, we all knew that the bottom often dropped off quite quickly along these sandbars. Mac, no doubt due to his fatigue, had forgotten about that. He emerged, grabbed his cap, and clawed his way up the steep sandbank, eliciting peals of laughter from his audience. Central Africans, as we have discussed, have a wonderful sense of humor and especially enjoy slapstick humor.

Mac had just blessed them with one of the most hilarious scenes that they had seen in ages. Mac, however, was not laughing.

We only almost died one time on the trip. There were some harrowing moments when our lumbering craft shot through narrows with impressive rapids, but we were safe enough with Joseph at the helm. The nearly fatal experience took place on a wide, peaceful-looking, lake-like, water-hyacinth-dotted expanse of the river. As we were paddling sedately across the flat-calm waters, a massive mother hippo broke the surface just a hundred yards or so off our starboard bow. Her baby trailed behind her. I will always remember the mother's eyes. These were eyes filled with pure hatred, and they were locked right onto us as she charged toward our canoe, pushing up a huge bow wake. Then she submerged and Joseph, having grown up on the river, knew that we were in grave danger. A mother hippo will do whatever it takes to protect her baby, and that includes both capsizing a 1,000-pound canoe and biting all of its occupants in half.

Joseph, who was usually quite calm, yelled, *"VITE! VITE! VITE!"* which is French for *Do as I say, or we will all die*. We got the message and dug with our paddles like our lives depended on it as Joseph steered us away from the hippo. That is, all of us except for Mac, who was in the bow, fumbling through his pack for the plastic bag containing his camera. He saw this as a perfect opportunity to get some action shots of African wildlife, once the hippo resurfaced. The poor guy had some unflattering comments directed his way, in three different languages, by all four of his crewmates, as we propelled our craft forward at a speed that would have made someone watching from shore assume we were fitted with an outboard motor. There was just something about anticipating being chomped in half that added an extra incentive to getting away quickly. Even Mac, once he detected the urgency in our profanity, put down his camera and contributed to the cause. I am certain that what saved us was Joseph's quick thinking and his ability to motivate us to convince the mother hippo that we were doing our best to distance ourselves from her baby.

Except for one close call with pirates, the last leg of our voyage was uneventful. As we were passing between the Zaire side of the river and a forested island, we unwittingly passed the hideout of some would-be pirates. Once our lumbering vessel was spotted, a small, fast-moving pirogue shot out from their lair. It was piloted by two unsavory types who saw us as easy white targets to board and plunder. The men who spend their lives paddling pirogues on the river develop an interesting physique. Their upper bodies resemble those of bodybuilders, while their legs look thin and atrophied. As they drew near, I could observe their physiques, but, more importantly, they could observe Mac's physique. They obviously had never encountered anyone as large or blond as Mac, so they turned their pirogue like a top and scooted back to their ambush spot as quickly as they had come. For that, we forgave Mac for almost getting us chomped in half by an enraged hippo.

By this time, we had resorted to drinking straight river water, since we were basically doing that already using Stewart's sand-filtration method. As we limped into the marina in Bangui, we were well loaded up with the more popular intestinal parasites. As a welcome to the capital, a group of fishermen stood around and distracted us while another one slipped around the pirogue and stole Stewart's pack, containing his clothes, camera, and sunscreen. We sold the pirogue to our director, since this was certainly a one-way canoe trip, got dewormed, had a few celebratory beers, and found rides back to our posts.

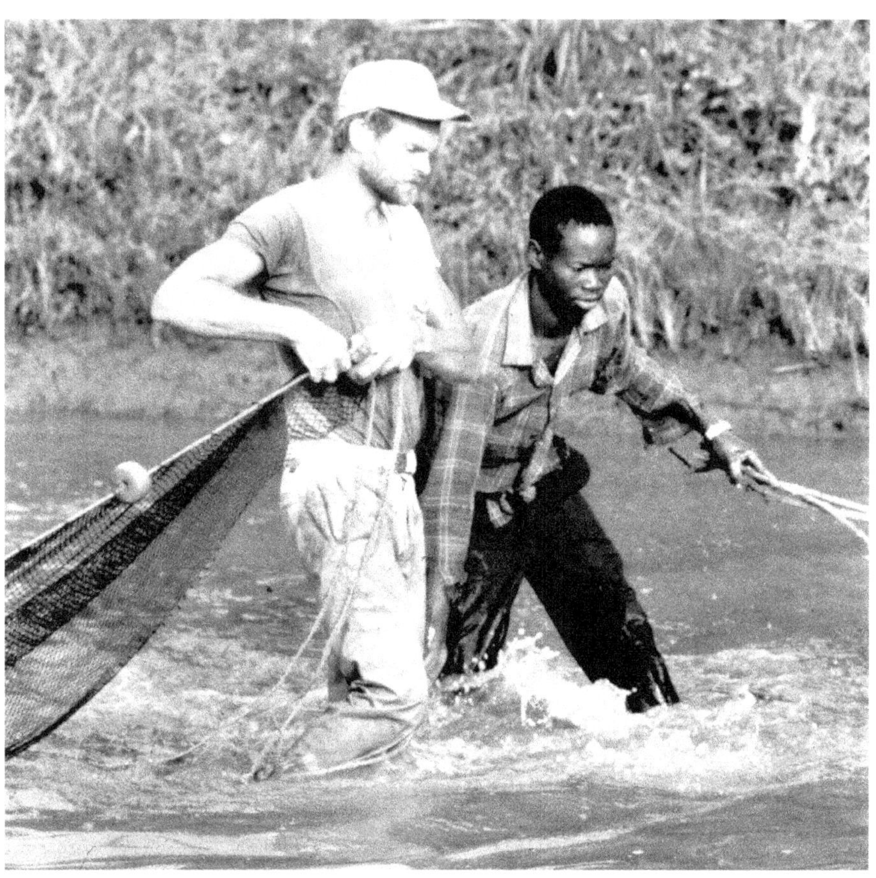

My final fish harvest at Oye' Carrefour before leaving Mobaye

TERMINATION

It is such a negative word, but *termination* was the word used to define the end of our Peace Corps service. It was not nearly as bad, though, as *early termination*, which meant leaving without fulfilling the pledges made during our swearing-in ceremony. Of the five of us, Mac and I were the only ones to terminate after completing our two years of service (plus some time tacked on for training new volunteers). Rebecca, Pete, and Tom all stayed for a third year. Tom then transferred to Malawi, where he served an additional two years. Pete is still in Africa, and is, as of this writing, the Director for USAID in Senegal. On our way home, Mac and I, along with two terminating teachers, camped out in Paris hostels for a couple of weeks, basically just eating and drinking.

I returned to Minnesota in late October, just in time for some prime duck, grouse, and deer hunting, which generated the pictures that so amazed Peg's friends back in Mobaye. I missed a fisheries position in northern Minnesota by a week, was strung along by another aquaculture venture that finally realized it had no money, and was facing the prospect of a winter back in my old bedroom in the basement of the house I grew up in. Few prospects can so stimulate action, so I responded to an ad in the back of an aquaculture magazine for a job working on a tropical fish farm in Lakeland, Florida. Raising aquarium fish is a world away from raising fish for food, but I did have fun breeding Oscars. Some of their practices, such as pouring pesticides into ponds to stress the fish, which stimulated brilliant colors, were disgusting.

So, when the call came from the University of Oklahoma, asking if I would be interested in being a trainer for a session of the Peace Corps Fisheries Program, I jumped at it. To top it off, Mac was to be one of the other trainers. It was loads of fun. By September of 1985, Peg was back at home. We got together, both for her to meet my parents in Minnesota, and for me to meet hers in New York. Then we really got together when we got married in November of 1986. For the next thirteen years, we lived in New York, Florida, and then back in New York.

Peg became a registered nurse while I worked in surface water management, aquaculture, water chemistry, and even served time as a school bus driver. What began as a two-year adventure to help land a job back in Bemidji ended up taking sixteen years. How much of that time was spent responding to nudges, and how much was spent defying them, is not entirely clear. But the moves that prompted the creation of my family were definitely responses to nudges. My father once said, "Dad should never have moved us from Iowa to northern Minnesota. That was a mistake." I responded, perhaps a bit selfishly, that since I would not be here if my grandfather had stayed in Iowa, I considered it a brilliant move.

If we stop to think about the infinite number of chance encounters between couples, going back countless generations, that led to our existence, it is as overwhelming as trying to make sense of the vastness of the universe. It is probably best to just accept our time here with gratitude and do our best to go about our lives with a grateful, contented spirit. A much more basic concept to grasp than infinity, and the one in 400 trillion odds (yes, it has been calculated) of us being *us*, is the realization that we need each other, and we need the natural world that sustains us. The Central African villagers got it. What better way to connect with each other than to share a good meal and time around the evening fire together?

SAUCE TOMATE

For those of you who made it to the end of this book (or skipped to the last page to see how it ends) I want to share with you a variation of my favorite meal in the CAR, Celestin's creation that is still one of our favorite meals. Although it is not quite the same without ripe-picked plantains, village-made palm oil, and hand-roasted and mashed peanuts, it is still a meal that transports us back to Mobaye. Even family and friends who would not be open to many of the meals we enjoyed in the CAR enjoy this meal and request the recipe.

About 4 servings

1 cup natural creamy peanut butter
½ cup coconut, palm, or olive oil
1–2 cloves garlic, minced or crushed
1 medium onion, diced
1 28-oz can of crushed tomatoes (or about 4 ripe tomatoes, diced)
½ lb. fresh spinach (or 10 oz of frozen spinach, thawed and drained)
2–3 ripe plantains
1 cup white rice
red pepper
salt

If rice is desired, first cook 1 cup of rice in about 2 cups of water, either in a rice cooker or on the stove top. (Rice is optional, in my opinion, as long as there are enough plantains.)

Heat ¼ cup of oil in a saucepan and add the diced onion. Cook over medium heat to soften the onion. Add the garlic and stir just a few seconds before adding the tomatoes. If using fresh tomatoes, stir and cook until softened.

Stir in the peanut butter. Depending on the consistency of the tomatoes, more peanut butter may be added to thicken the sauce. Stir in a pinch of red pepper.

Stir in the spinach and cook until it is wilted. Meanwhile, heat the other ¼ cup of olive oil in a large frying pan. Peel the plantains, cut them in half, and cut each half lengthwise. Fry the quarters in oil over low-medium heat until they become lightly browned on one side. Flip them and brown the other side. Taste the sauce to determine if it needs salt. Adjust the salt and hot pepper amounts to suit your taste.

The sauce is served over the plantains (and the rice, if you opt to cook rice). Like most good recipes, this one is to be used as a guideline. Experienced or confident cooks generally adapt a recipe to suit their tastes and to the ingredients available. I seldom make this dish the same way twice. In season, we like to use our own fresh tomatoes and spinach. If we don't have spinach, we use swiss chard. Plantains are never in season in northern Minnesota, of course, so we make do with what we can get. It may not be Celestin's *sauce tomate*, but it is always a reasonable substitute for it.

Bon Appetit!

MERCI

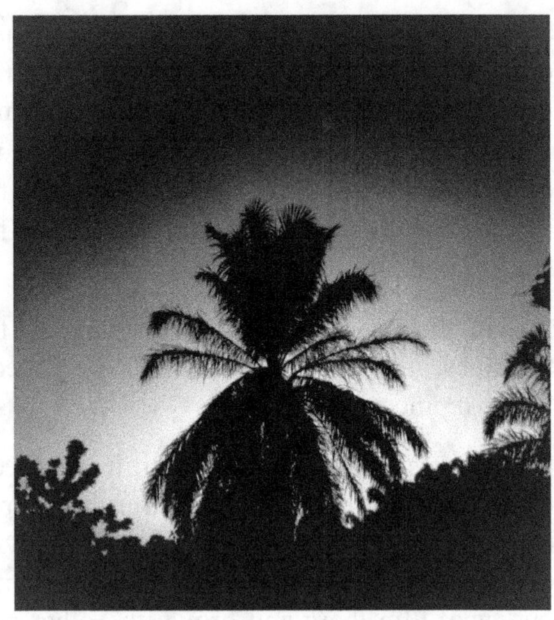

We lost Tom Fondell to pancreatic cancer in 2017. Thankfully, Peg and I, along with Rebecca and her husband, Jay (also a CAR volunteer), and Tom's wife, Melonie were blessed with a few days together at Tom's brother's lake cabin in Minnesota, in October of 2016. We ate gloriously (including Sauce Tomate), shared fond memories, and parted with lots of hugs and some poorly concealed tears. I have Tom to thank, not only for giving me some great stories to share with my grandson, but for being instrumental in keeping me in the CAR long enough to meet Peggy. Basse Kotto Boy #1 is sorely missed.

I am also grateful to the agents and fish farmers, as well as the Central African villagers in general, for reminding me about what is most important in life. I think of them, and of the beautiful ponds that we created, often. In my dreams they are still teeming with tilapia.

Many thanks to Heather Johnson of *Garden of Edits* for her excellent command of the English language, which made my stories, if not more believable, then at least more readable.

I must thank my wife, Peggy, for her unconditional love and support. Had her love been conditional, I would have been in deep trouble long ago. It is only through her unwavering support of my dreams (and her ability to bankroll them), that I have been able to pursue them. Since a good share of those dreams would have been better left in the dream stage, I am grateful.

I also must thank Conor and Sarah, who, besides being my valuable resident critics, had to endure several failed endeavors that I am sure left you sometimes wondering what it must be like growing up with a normal dad. But I do believe that teaching our children to appreciate and prefer whole, real food is one of the greatest gifts that a parent can give to their children. It would thrill me to no end if you someday say to your own children: Just eat how your parents eat, and all will be well. You have big hearts, and that makes mine feel quite content.

ABOUT THE AUTHOR

Mark Schultz operates a business in Bemidji, Minnesota called *Backwood Basics*. His passion for gardening, hunting & fishing, sailing, canoeing, and well-prepared meals, has inspired him to develop products and ideas to help others nurture a more self-reliant lifestyle. His time spent in the heart of Africa taught him many life lessons about being content with what we have, as well as gaining a deep respect for the natural world that sustains us.

www.ingramcontent.com/pod-product-compliance
Lightning Source LLC
Chambersburg PA
CBHW050728260726
48661CB00001B/112